THE NURSE AS WOUNDED HEALER:
FROM TRAUMA TO TRANSCENDENCE

Marion Conti-O'Hare

THE NURSE AS WOUNDED HEALER:

From Trauma to Transcendence

Marion Conti-O'Hare, PhD, RN, CS, HNC

JONES AND BARTLETT PUBLISHERS
Sudbury, Massachusetts
BOSTON   TORONTO   LONDON   SINGAPORE

World Headquarters
Jones and Bartlett Publishers
40 Tall Pine Drive
Sudbury, MA 01776
978-443-5000

Jones and Bartlett Publishers Canada
2406 Nikanna Road
Mississauga, ON L5C 2W6
CANADA

Jones and Bartlett Publishers International
Barb House, Barb Mews
London W6 7PA
UK

Library of Congress Cataloging-in-Publication Data
Conti-O'Hare, Marion.
    The nurse as wounded healer : from trauma to transcendence /
Marion Conti-O'Hare.
       p.; cm.
    Includes bibliographical references and index.
    ISBN: 0-7637-1568-9
       1. Nurses—Psychology. 2. Nursing—Philosophy. I. Title.
    [DNLM: 1. Nurses—psychology. 2. Philosophy, Nursing. 3. Stress,
    Psychological—psychology. WY 87 C762n 2002]
    RT86 .C665 2002
    610.73'01'9—dc21
                                                        2002029708

Production Credits
Acquisitions Editor: Penny M. Glynn
Associate Editor: Christine Tridente
Production Editor: Anne Spencer
Editorial Assistant: Thomas Prindle
Manufacturing Buyer: Amy Duddridge
Cover Design: Anne Spencer
Cover Image: © 2001 Alex Grey. *Journey of the Wounded Healer, panel #3.*
    www.alexgrey.com
Design and Composition: Carlisle Communications, Ltd.
Printing and Binding: Malloy Lithographing

Printed in the United States of America
07 06 05 04 03   10 9 8 7 6 5 4 3 2

ABOUT THE AUTHOR

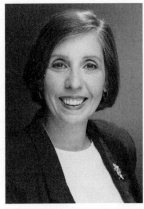

Marion Conti-O'Hare has practiced in the field of psychiatric/mental health nursing for over 17 years. She received a B.A. in psychology from St. Joseph's College, Patchogue, N.Y., a B.S. in nursing from S.U.N.Y. at Stony Brook, an M.S.N. from Sacred Heart University, Fairfield, Conn., an M.S. in Community Mental Health Counseling from Long Island University, Greenvale, N.Y., and a Ph.D. from Adelphi University, Garden City, N.Y. At present, she holds certification as a holistic nurse, addictions registered nurse, clinical specialist in psychiatric/mental health nursing, and is a New York state credentialed alcoholism and substance abuse counselor.

Dr. Conti-O'Hare has served as adjunct professor at New York University and Adelphi University and as consultant to the New York College for Wholistic Health Education and Research. In addition, she has presented papers at national and international conferences on such topics as the nurse's therapeutic use of self and on holistic nursing theory and practice. She has also published in these areas.

The founder of Personal Wellness Consultation, a holistic nursing practice, Dr. Conti-O'Hare seeks to help health care professionals promote their own well-being.

Making one's own wounds a source of healing requires the constant willingness to see one's own pain and suffering as rising from the depth of the human condition which all people share.

~Henry J. M. Nouwen, *The Wounded Healer*

About the Cover

JOURNEY OF THE WOUNDED HEALER

After a profound transformation, the wounded healer, "a reintegrated man ascends into the middle and upper worlds, released from the psychic bonds of materialistic entrapment and tapped into the light which beams from the mind and heart. As a healer, he wields a crystalline hermetic caduceus with the balanced serpent powers of the unconscious and winged version of the superconscious. The healer/scientist/artist ascends the crystal mountain of the higher self, a self empowered by the responsibility for healing the future."

~Grey, A. (1990). *Sacred mirrors: The visionary art of Alex Grey.* Rochester, VT: Inner Traditions International.

PREFACE

As members of the healing professions, nurses have traditionally been viewed as caretakers and, as such, bring their own experiences to the work setting. With caring, compassion, and empathy as the basic components of nursing, we are expected to practice these values in furthering the healing process. When personal or professional wounding has occurred, it will undoubtedly be manifested in our contacts with peers, students, patients, and the public. If untreated, wounds persist as remnants of developmental trauma, and our inadequate efforts to cope with them may lead to addictions or dysfunctional relationships.

In some circles, experts allude to the fragility of nursing and perceive it as a wounded profession. No more clearly has this been demonstrated than in the inability of nurses to have a significant voice in crucial national and international health care policies. The problem has been exacerbated by a rapidly changing health care environment, which chastises them for becoming more impersonal and mechanized. Furthermore, the profession exists within a health care system undergoing severe wounding. As a result nursing's contributions have been minimized, intensifying the pain of its practitioners.

Prior to the events of 9/11/01, the need for healing had already assumed marked importance with the prevalence of violence on the national and international scene. More frequent and shocking incidents of shootings by children and youth produced a wake-up call to the American public searching for answers. A growing awareness emerged, reflecting the need for meaning in the lives of people, particularly among the alienated and disconnected, those unable to cope often resorting to destructive or antisocial acts.

After the terrorist attacks in the United States, however, trauma descended upon a nation and the world, destroying our innocence. The horror of that September morning left emotional scars that are not easily forgotten on almost all feeling people. Since trauma has a cumulative effect and does not resolve itself, the resulting hurt becomes a deterrent to addressing the pain and prevents effective healing. As a result, the walking wounded now abound on our planet.

Acquiring more knowledge about trauma is critical to the nursing community as it strives to understand itself and those for whom it provides service and care. Nurses have been portrayed as *wounded healers*, but precisely what this means has not been explored in any depth within the profession. Who actually can be called a "wounded healer," and what are the manifestations of this calling? Perhaps there is a more compelling question: *Can a profession survive that does not heal itself?*

Although the terms *wounding* and *healing* appear to reflect separate and antithetical notions, combining the two into a single unified concept, that of the "wounded healer," can potentially generate some remarkable outcomes in health care. Healers are expected to attend to people wounded spiritually, emotionally, or physically—or a combination of all three. There is evidence to support the theory that a person who has endured trauma becomes a more successful healer. At the same time, is it fair to assume that healers who have not experienced serious wounding are unable to facilitate the healing process as successfully?

The central thrust of this book is to provide for the first time an examination of the nurse as a wounded healer and its effect on the practice of nursing. It describes how healing has been defined in the past, and emphasizes the changing focus necessary to meet the relevant health care needs of an increasingly wounded society. Beginning with an historical perspective, the work describes healing practices of ancient civilizations, the numerous types of healers and how they function, the theories employed, and the roots and repercussions of the traumatic experience. Each step in the healing process has been delineated leading to reflection and from there to transformation and transcendence.

Also proposed is an innovative model for practitioners to follow. A major feature that appears in later sections of the book includes fascinating vignettes of people in fact and fiction who became wounded healers, including nurses and nonnurses. Targeted to nursing educators, practitioners, and students as well as other professionals, the work serves as a useful resource to help nurses articulate the nature of their trauma, facilitate healing of their own woundedness, and become more vocal in healing their profession.

Marion Conti-O'Hare

ACKNOWLEDGMENTS

It is a privilege to acknowledge some of the people who contributed generously their time and expertise to the preparation of this work. I am deeply grateful to my husband John and our two daughters Anne and Patricia, whose patience and encouragement helped to move the book along.

For their ongoing support, I am indebted to my colleagues, Dr. Elvira Miller, Associate Director for Patient Services, Department of Veterans Affairs, New York Harbor Health Care System, and to Janet Bezmen-Idema, Associate Executive Director for Psychiatry, Elmhurst Hospital, N.Y.

In particular, I extend my gratitude to the members of Nursing Program VIII as well as Mary Ellen Mungovan, Nora O'Hanlon, and Joan Kendrew at the New York College for Wholistic Health Education and Research. Their healing spirit continues to sustain me.

Finally, I wish to express my appreciation to Dr. Shirley Fondiller, whose knowledge, wise counsel, and superb editorial skill guided me throughout the effort from inception to completion.

Foreword

This book is an invitation as well as an invocation to nurses to evolve into the healers they are, although the process may not be possible without honoring the wounded healer phenomenon. The author breaks new ground, revealing that practitioners, educators, students, and patients demonstrate their own healing nature by experiencing and confronting their past, present, and future as a vignette of living one's woundedness. Implicit in this observation is acknowledging that the wounds that hurt are also those which heal. By recognizing the causes and consequences of trauma in our lives, nurses and other health professionals can become the healers they are destined to be. Such an awakening affirms our humanity as we connect and transform. When shared, the wounds emanating from a traumatic episode can foster self-revelation and ignite the potential for developing as mature individuals and health care practitioners. In this seminal work, Marion Conti-O'Hare aptly points out that the willingness to enter into new territory and successfully transcend the wounded space that we all inhabit enables us to expand the human condition and our common healing processes.

Jean M. Watson, Ph.D., RN, FAAN
Distinguished Professor
Endowed Chair in Caring Science
Center of Human Caring
University of Colorado
Denver, Colorado, 80262 USA

CONTENTS

PART I

INTRODUCTION

With the plethora of literature dealing with the topic of healing, it is easy to think that nothing else could be new. A false assumption? Indeed yes, in light of modern science and technological innovations that have altered dramatically the way we think, feel, work, and live. Everyday we read in the newspaper or see on television, new ways to foster healing. Consider the progress under way relating to regenerative medicine designed to eliminate disease and extend life. According to researchers in the field, healing the body will no longer depend on scalpels and medications, but on the cells and chemical signals that the human body uses to repair itself (Wade, 2000, p. F1).

Although these developments may seem mind-boggling, certain fundamental values relating to the healing phenomenon have endured over the centuries and continue to affect the human condition: We can point to various cultures, in which caring, curing, and healing have remained constants over time, even with shifts occurring in emphasis and direction.

Some health professionals equate curing with healing, and unwittingly use the terms interchangeably, but both represent different concepts. "Curing," which comes from the Latin *cura*, focuses on recovery or relief from a disease and reflects cause and effect, and finality. On the other hand, "healing" is derived from the English *hal*, which means "to make whole," and usually is used in reference to some type of injury or wounding that can be physical, psychological, or social in nature (Keegan, 1994).

Although healers can be defined simplistically as people who heal, the methods they employ differ markedly. Practitioners who assume that certain healing practices are superior to others may be promulgating dangerous attitudes that lead to deleterious consequences. Authentic healers base interventions on the needs of their patients rather than their own, an approach requiring openness and honesty on the part of the nurse. Thirty years ago

1

when the holistic movement took hold, its leaders confined their practice primarily to the use of herbs, massage, and natural remedies, but over the next two decades they broadened their focus, based on an expanding awareness of the need to integrate or combine methods appropriate for the individual patient (Weil, 1983). The evolution of holistic nursing stemmed from the dissatisfaction of the nursing community with Western medicine.

According to McKivergin (1999), the healing process involves an exchange of energy, truth, and communication between nurses and their patients to "help them attune to their own healing capacities and implement the healthiest response for any given situation" (p. 209). Wendler (1996) perceives healing as a more global phenomenon than curing and urges nurses to examine healing not only in regard to patients but also in reference to themselves. Unfortunately, this aspect of the therapeutic relationship evokes discomfort in many practitioners.

Some authorities, such as Montgomery-Dossey & Guzzetta (2000), claim that healing represents a return to the natural state of integrity and the individual's wholeness. A process evolves in which certain aspects of the self, body, mind, and spirit are interconnected at a deep level of knowing from within that produces integration and balance, with each part achieving equal importance. The ultimate outcome results in more complex levels of personal understanding and meaning.

When people who have experienced wounding develop sound insights into their own situations, they are in a better position to communicate human warmth, which in turn helps patients heal (McGlone, 1990). All too often, however, health professionals are reluctant to reveal themselves because of the potential for vulnerability, created largely by an orientation toward perfection and flawless performance. Watson (1999) alludes to wounding in a larger context, noting that if nursing is to be "an expression of healing for self, others, and the culture of our health systems, we need to make our wounds conscious" (p. 30).

The process of recovery from a traumatic event requires a voyage of discovery in human development. Along the continuum, wounded healers may feel pain, seclude themselves, or resort to addictive behaviors. As nurses know, the core of their practice lies in the therapeutic use of self, which is the key to healing. How effectively they perform as healers relates closely to their beliefs and self-understanding.

An important factor applicable to the wounded healer concerns the degree of awareness of his or her own trauma and how it can be integrated into the relationship between the healer and the person to be healed. It is this recognition along with the willingness to accept and transcend one's own woundedness that sets the stage for generating true healing in others.

REFERENCES

Keegan, L. (1994). The nurse as healer. Albany, NY: Delmar.

McGlone, M. E. (1990). Healing the spirit. Holistic Nursing Practice, 4 (4), 77–84.

McKivergin, M. (1999). The nurse as an instrument of healing. In B. Montgomery-Dossey, L. Keegan, & C. E. Guzzetta (Eds.), Holistic nursing: A handbook for practice. (3rd ed., pp. 207–227). Gaithersberg, MD: Aspen.

Montgomery-Dossey, B., & Guzzeta, C. E. (2000). Holistic nursing practice. In B. Montgomery-Dossey, L. Keegan & C. E. Guzzeta (Eds.), Holistic nursing: A handbook for practice (3rd ed., pp. 5–33). Gaithersberg, MD: Aspen.

Wade, N. (2000, November 7). Teaching the body to heal itself. The New York Times, pp. F1, F8.

Watson, J. (1999). Postmodern nursing and beyond. New York: Churchill Livingstone.

Weil, A. (1983). Health and healing: Understanding conventional and alternative medicine. Boston: Houghton Mifflin.

Wendler, M. C. (1996). Understanding healing: A conceptual analysis. Journal of Advanced Nursing, 24, 836–842.

CHAPTER 1

HEALING PRACTICES THROUGH THE AGES: MYTHS, MAGIC, AND SUPERSTITION

A long time ago, man and animal lived together in peace and harmony. Suddenly this changed when some greedy people began to hunt only to sell the meat and fur. This caused the animal population to dwindle, greatly concerning the animals.

The white bear then called a council of their members to decide on how to avenge themselves. The oldest and wisest flies offered a suggestion: "Let us call upon the spirits." We will ask them to send great sickness on the people, and we will carry the diseases."

Eventually, a great sickness spread indeed through the Native American villages. Since the animals only wanted to punish the bad people, they were saddened to see the good ones suffering as well. They called another council to discuss what was to be done.

A solution came from the lowly herbs who promised to heal the sick. Then, spirit dreams were sent to the Shamans to guide them to the herbs. This is how healing medicine was brought to the Native American.

M. F. Lindemans, *The Coming of Medicine, Encyclopedia Mythica*

The concept of the wounded healer has conjured up a variety of imaginative and enigmatic notions, not the least being that it is a modern phenomenon. Such observations suggest some legitimacy that can be attributed, in part, to the increasing attention to healing practices, particularly those in the alternative or nontraditional realm. In fact, the wounded healer represents a complex entity of ancient lineage that continues to exert a marked impact on American life.

Although the art of healing has existed throughout the ages, with many of the practices well known, history does not always reveal the nature and motivations of the healers themselves. The data may be scarce, unavailable, or inadequate as in ancient times, since tablets, monuments, and other relics may not suffice. When observing the interaction between a healer and the person being healed, can we assume that the treatment's effectiveness depends largely on the dynamics of the relationship between the two and extends beyond the type of method employed? In this respect, does the healer who has suffered an earlier wounding have a greater capability for engendering a more successful outcome?

Although members of the health professions tend to relate their healing prowess to the health care milieu, the process encompasses a much broader universe. We have only to look at remarkable figures of the past like Eleanor Roosevelt and a modern hero such as Nelson Mandela. Both endured deep trauma in their lives and transcended it to the extent of healing nations in serious turmoil. What about the extraordinary Helen Keller, deaf and blind from childhood, whose humanitarian writings and lectures inspired people around the world?

Wounded healers are ubiquitous, although much lesser known than those cited above. This may be truer in the nursing profession than in other fields because of the very nature of the discipline and its expectations. We may even claim Florence Nightingale as a wounded healer, speculating whether her drive and determination to nurse in the Crimea might have been influenced by familial trauma. At the same time, there can be no doubt that the healing capacities of nurses like Mary Breckinridge and Margaret Sanger, whose vision sparked lasting causes, stemmed from enduring painful experiences during their young adult years.

A journey into the past to examine healing practices through the ages, represents a sound beginning in helping us address challenging questions and uncover new information. Exploring the intricacies that characterize wounded healers, including their patterns of behavior, can create fresh insights into advancing nursing in its various health care arenas.

NURSING AND HEALING: FROM ANTIQUITY TO CONTEMPORARY PRACTICE

The role of the nurse emerged as an intuitive response to a need for caring and healing in individuals and communities (Dolan, Fitzpatrick, & Hermann, 1983). From the beginning of civilization, human beings have instinctively wanted to protect, comfort, and nourish their offspring, with the mother viewed as the first nurse, "a warm, loving presence symbolizing security and warmth" (Masson, 1985, p. 13). The term "nurse" has a simple and noble origin, derived from the Latin words *nutrire* meaning "to nourish" and *nutrix* meaning "nursing mother."

In ancient times, people attributed illness to three major factors: a foreign body which caused pain and discomfort, deities venting their anger, or enemies trying to dispose of them. To eradicate the cause of their ailments, primitive people turned to the shaman or medicine man, perceived as someone having mysterious powers, who "could bargain with the dark powers on his behalf" (Masson, 1985, p. 13).

As the shaman's female counterpart, the medicine woman came into being, acting as midwife, nurse, and wise woman. She selected and prepared herbal concoctions, applied spider webs to sores, made grass plasters, and sucked and licked wounds. Through archeological excavations, striking evidence was unearthed about the healing methods employed by these early practitioners. Images of the female fertility goddesses revealed them to be the main icons of worship as well as sources of wisdom and healing powers. As the central deities, the goddesses provided knowledge of herbal remedies and poisons as well as interpretations of dreams for divination and diagnosis (Achterberg, 1991).

Dating back to 4000 B.C., the Sumerians emerged as the major influence for healing systems that developed throughout the world. Along the trade routes, theories of body function and disease spread to ancient Phoenicia, Greece, and Rome. In addition to surgery, herbal medications were selected from an extensive listing of ingredients that soothed, disinfected, and aided healing (Achterberg, 1991). From the Sumerian culture, similar therapies sprang up among civilizations whose health goals aimed to achieve a wholeness with the healing of the mind, body, and spirit. As a dominant force of the times, religion was linked to the healing practices performed by priests, shamans, and priestesses until approximately the third millennium before Christianity. An aura of magic and superstition was pervasive, with evil spirits viewed as the cause of illness. In such a climate, incantations, surgical procedures, and potions flourished to rid the body of disease and demons (Dolan, Fitzpatrick, & Hermann, 1983).

Of interest is that although indigenous societies perceived the supernatural to be involved in illness and healing, their approach to maintaining health was holistic in nature. Native Americans, for example, espoused the need for balance among mankind, nature, and the supernatural. They introduced their own plant medicines, sweat baths, gentle massage, and other types of body manipulation. These early healers offered an amazing variety of methods or techniques to be applied in the healing process.

Porter (1997) describes the practices of the Amerindians as using sassafras, holly, and sunflowers, along with inhaling the smoke from burning twigs, to treat chest congestion. Another popular practice was "blowing on the sick," in which the breath and the laying on of hands would purge the infirmity (p. 164). Curiously, the people were not subjected to a wide range of diseases until they began to domesticate animals and until foreign explorers transmitted a host of illnesses brought from their native lands.

The ancient traditions of Chinese medicine assume marked importance in light of their application to modern-day healing methods. Thousands of years before the advent of Christianity, the Chinese performed healing by treating disharmonies in health. Their goal was to assist individuals in acquiring balance, higher functional status, and a transcendence of illness. They considered human beings to be a "microcosm of the universe as part of an unbroken wholeness" (Beinfield & Korngold, 1991).

Within Chinese tradition, nature was seen as a unified energy system, or Tao, that consisted of polar and complementary opposites known as Yin and Yang, which interdependently organized the universe. Whereas Yin reflected substance, darkness, quietness, cold, inertia, and death, Yang represented form, light, noise, warmth, activity, and birth (Beinfield & Korngold, 1991). When a balance occurred between the two components, health emerged as the outcome.

The Chinese believed that healing could be accomplished by determining long-standing patterns of imbalance between Yin and Yang. They treated physical, mental, or spiritual deviations with combinations of body work, acupuncture, and herbs. Other popular methods included hydrotherapy, cupping (bleeding), cauterizing, and systematic exercise (Kelly & Joel, 1995).

Espousing a philosophical view similar to that of the Chinese, India introduced a medical system called Ayurveda, which aimed to be consonant with harmonies of the universe and religious teachings (Porter, 1997). Staying healthy required temperance in all matters, especially in regard to food, sleep, exercise, sexual practices, and even prescribed medications. Washing, diets, and exercise regimens were practiced according to the Hindu belief in rebirth, renunciation, and maintaining balance of the soul. In addition to the application of herbs, treatments included ointments, enemas, douches, massage, sweats, and surgery (Porter, 1997).

Among African societies, the belief prevailed that health was achieved when the individual experienced self-harmony. In various communities, female members performed the role of nurses while the shamans or witch doctors practiced medical functions. Their treatment consisted of the extensive use of herbal remedies and potions. The ceremonial procedures involving healing reflected unity between physical, emotional, and spiritual factors, stimulating families and communities to participate in singing, dancing, and other musical rituals (Dolan, Fitzpatrick, & Hermann, 1983).

In other parts of the world such as Egypt, specialized clergy or physicians were responsible for treating disease. Endowed with their own hierarchy and rules, they practiced a mixture of magic and empiricism based on some knowledge of anatomy, pharmacology, and pathology (Ghalioungui, 1963). Their ministrations, which relied on homeopathy, charms, spells, and prayer, were also closely intertwined with the religious system of gods and goddesses. It was not unusual for a physician to pray over a medicine before giving it to the affected person (Ghalioungui, 1963).

Egyptian physicians revealed a uniqueness by their gentle and meticulous approach to treating patients. Unlike other cultures, in which the sick were often considered untouchables, their performance reflected a humane attitude. Nowhere was this more clearly demonstrated than in the work of Imhotep, who introduced the practice of embalming, classified 250 diseases, and developed drugs and the treatment required for care (Doheny, Cook, & Stopper, 1982). Following his death, Egypt honored him as a god.

Among others practicing the healing arts were the queens of Egypt including Mentuhotep, Hatsheput, and Cleopatra (Masson, 1985). Of particular interest were the Egyptian nurses of the newborn, named after Hathor, the goddess who protected infants. Their role involved helping the development of the Ka, or nonobservable replica of the body representing the source of all attributes and delimitations of the physical body such as illness (Krieger, 1981, p. 64). All these advances, however, did not eliminate magic and ritualistic practices which persisted for some time.

In describing the origins of people along with their health, illnesses, and medical practices, perhaps no source was more revealing than the stories emanating from Greek mythology with fascinating tales exhalting the ruling gods and goddesses. Imbued with many gifts, Apollo became the deity closely associated with healing, and his son, Asclepios, the god of medicine, acquired his knowledge from Chiron, the wisest of all centaurs, who is believed to be the original model of the wounded healer. Half man, half horse, Chiron had received an incurable, crippling wound which forced him into a life of chronic pain and suffering; yet he developed the capability of healing others and ultimately transcended his own wounding.

During the thirteenth century B.C., Asclepios earned some prominence as the architect of the exquisitely decorated healing temples, located in areas of natural beauty and fed by spring water. Functioning as health resorts, these sanctuaries offered therapeutic regimens that encompassed mainly diets and exercise, but also included mineral springs, baths, gymnasiums, and athletic fields as well as treatment and consultation rooms (Kelly & Joel, 1995). Among the female deities dominating healing in the Greco-Roman world were Hygeia, daughter of Asclepios; Artemis, goddess of the woods; and Isis, the Egyptian goddess mother. Hygeia became known as the first and most powerful healing deity (Abrahamsen, 1997), as reflected in an ancient hymn:

Queen of all, charming and lovely and blooming
Blessed Hygeia, mother of all, bringer of prosperity, hear me
Through you vanish the diseases that afflict us,
and through you every house blossoms to the fullness of joy
and the arts thrive (Reis, 1991, pp. 162–163).

One of the most important practices associated with cures was the incubation ritual, or "temple sleep," in which afflicted people were housed within a sacred enclosure. Under such conditions, which could span from one day up to several weeks, the supplicants believed in the deities as performing the actual healing or appearing in dreams to prescribe the proper treatment (Abrahamsen, 1997). A rather chilling example occurred in the case of Arata, a Spartan woman who had dropsy. Her mother had left her at home and had gone to the Temple of Asclepios to pray for her recovery. There, she dreamed that a god decapitated the daughter, hung her upside down, and then placed her head back on the body. Upon returning to Sparta, she discovered that Arata had experienced the same dream and was cured (Lefkowitz & Fant, 1982).

Vast numbers of supplicants flocked to these medical shrines hoping to be healed by the miraculous interventions of the gods (Scarborough, 1969). As religious institutions controlled by priests, the healing temples consisted of a routine of prayer, sacrifices, rituals, and grateful offerings such as money, artwork, statues, or figurines to honor the gods (Abrahamsen, 1997).

In the annals of Greek thought, as new attitudes began to evolve, changes occurred in the society that gradually affected healing practices. A dominant contributor to the process was the physician and scholar Hippocrates (circa 460–370 B.C.), who introduced the concept of rational or scientific medicine. He theorized that the breaking of nature's laws caused disease rather than the accepted belief that demons, spirits, or gods were the culprits. Known as the Father of Medicine, Hippocrates viewed the helping role of the physician as one that would foster healing by addressing the health of the entire body and not merely a particular organ or part. He also emphasized the need to understand the patient's environment as well as the presenting symptoms of an illness.

According to Hippocrates, health depended on a state of equilibrium among various internal factors governing the operations of the body and mind. He believed that this equilibrium could be attained only when man lived in harmony with his external environment (Dolan, Fitzpatrick, & Hermann, 1983). The great philosopher Plato succinctly summed up this holistic approach by stating that "to heal even an eye, one must heal the head, even the whole body" (p. 35).

Many of the healing and medical practices stemming from ancient Greece were adapted by the Romans who embellished the therapeutic spas and introduced new treatment modalities. The famous baths, named after the emperor Diocletian, housed over 3,000 rooms. The services provided to patrons involved massage, followed by what could be characterized as the prototype of the modern sauna. Hot and cold water immersion completed the treatment designed to cleanse the mind, body, and spirit (Keegan, 1994).

Through the writings of Galen, a Greek physician born in the early Christian era (circa 130 A.D.), Hippocratic principles were employed during the reign of the Roman Empire. His prodigious work addressed the physical sciences and described at least 473 drugs of various types. He also encouraged sea voyages, moderate exercise, sun exposure, massage, and warm baths (Dolan, Fitzpatrick, & Hermann, 1983).

Although Galen's contributions accelerated the evolution of scientific medicine, traditional healing practices continued. Slaves or former slaves, as well as other types of healers, began to appear along with body builders, root gatherers, and others not always perceived as reputable (Porter, 1997). Self-help activities became universal including written guides for surgical and other healing methods available to the public. In spite of the mystical or supernatural views of illness that persisted, the Roman Empire produced remarkable advances in environmental conditions, most notably sanitation and sewage facilities to improve public health.

THE MIDDLE AGES:
IMPACT OF WOMEN HEALERS

The advent of Christianity ushered in different approaches toward healing and health, particularly through the changing role of women as primary healers. With the passing of the medicine women in ancient cultures, nurses began to lose their status and some of their civil rights. They were often relegated to a lower social position in their work, suffering discrimination and sometimes death in a slave economy (Dolan, Fitzpatrick, & Hermann, 1983). Nurses practiced primarily as midwives or as caregivers for women and children; they continued to use folk measures for healing and the laying on of hands. Eventually, however, the physician's orders directed nursing practice.

Perhaps the narrow domain accorded to nurses or women in the health field can be best illustrated in the early Greek legend involving Agnodice and the extent to which she went to practice medicine. Distressed by the anguish of women who preferred death to being examined by a man, this courageous Athenian woman cross-dressed in an effort to study and serve as a healer. Agnodice eventually became a symbol to other women who sought medical education during the nineteenth century (Porter, 1997).

In the middle ages, female healers began to flourish. Most notable was Hildegarde of Bingen (1098–1179), whose book on medicine dealt with the healing powers of herbs, stones, and animals, as well as other methods. In medieval times, institutions began to open up to care for the sick, along with religious orders operated by deaconesses. These women—who could be viewed as forerunners of the modern community or visiting nurse—provided basic care to the needy and the ill. They relied primarily on home remedies using herbs, minerals, diets, baths, and fresh air (Porter, 1997).

With their eventual dissolution, the deaconesses were replaced by a group of nurses higher in social status. Roman matrons of wealthy lineage showed great interest in nursing and, after converting to Christianity, initiated efforts to help the community to promote health practices. Elevated to sainthood for their caring work were such illustrious figures as Lady Marcella, Lady Paula, and Lady Fabiola (Dolan, Fitzpatrick, & Hermann, 1983).

During the Middle Ages, nursing became more organized into military, religious, and secular orders (Doheny, Cook, & Stopper, 1982). At the time of the Crusades, from the eleventh through the thirteenth centuries, the Knights Hospitallers represented the first military order of nurses. In addition, three other orders of knights were established to tend and protect the wounded. Although dominated by men, some women were in active service, but they were permitted to work only in hospitals and to care for other women (Kelly & Joel, 1995).

Although religion remained the dominant force in nursing, a visible group of lay women healers came into prominence. Generally portrayed as individuals from the lower classes, they became known as "wise women" or "witches" who traveled to villages and homes to service the poor and the infirm. Because of restrictions preventing them from studying medicine in the university, the information they acquired depended on tradition and folklore. They employed a host of effective remedies tested by years of use, such as digitalis for heart conditions and belladonna for use as an antispasmodic.

The healing practices of the witches became a threat to physicians as well as to the Catholic Church, which catered to the ruling class that cultivated the university-prepared doctor. As empiricists, witches relied on their senses, trial and error, and cause and effect, rather than on faith or religious doctrine. In one respect, their "magic" was the science of the times. Accused of such heinous acts as murder and poisoning, along with sexual crimes, they were hanged or burned at the stake in large numbers. Significantly, the persecution of witches did not stem from the methods used but rather from the political bias toward women (Ehenreich & English, 1973). Although witch hunting gradually declined and death penalties were abolished in some European countries, a belief in the power of the witches persisted into the late 1700s.

The Renaissance of the sixteenth century furthered the scientific method of inquiry, generating advances in the medical profession and emphasizing the importance of gaining knowledge about various healing modalities including surgery and medicine. Approaches to self-help sprang up with the invention of the printing press, which enabled the dissemination of health care information to the public. People learned how to monitor their health while they gleaned advice on such topics as healthful location of the home, organizing a household, and eating and drinking, and exercise tips (Porter, 1997).

The growth of anatomical knowledge and its application to surgery gave increased recognition to the need for educated nurses. Subsequently, the Sisters of Charity, a nursing order in France, offered one of the first programs to prepare selected nuns with high ideals and standards. Along with a spiritual focus, their nursing practice involved a wide range of skills including the use of drugs and simple surgical procedures (Porter, 1997).

A significant feature of the Renaissance was the division created in the Church that led to the Protestant Reformation. As interest in religion and church support waned and as monasteries closed, a "dark period" in health care emerged and continued into the mid-nineteenth century. In contrast to the earlier charitable institutions based on spiritual faith and healing intention, public institutions deteriorated. Bare, dark, and poorly ventilated, they resembled prisons more than hospitals (Keegan, 1994). Nursing became secularized, lost its status, and was considered a "last resort occupation" for women (Doheny, Cook, & Stopper, 1982, p. 54). Dickens' graphic description of the notorious Sairy Gamp and Betsy Prig exemplified the types of women who performed nursing at that time. He purposely wrote about these characters to warn the public about the dangers of allowing unqualified persons to care for the sick.

CHANGING MEDICAL AND NURSING HEALING PRACTICES

A turning point in the history of healing can be traced to the period between the sixteenth and seventeenth centuries when Descartes formulated his theory related to the separation of mind and body. Guided by this model, healing strategies began to stress the view that human beings could be understood and controlled if they were conceived of as machines (Porter, 1997). This dehumanizing approach led to a belief in reductionism and the advent of modern-day medical science.

Although most earlier healing systems had emphasized the relationship of the sick person to the wider universe, Western medicine adopted a more limited perspective with the body seen solely as the dominant focus (Porter, 1997). In the wake of Cartesian dualism, a dramatic shift from holistic to reductionistic thought occurred, and the goal of treatment focused on curing rather than on a balance between individual and environmental factors. This development contributed to the polarization of caring and curing in the healing arts (Achterberg, 1991).

During the late eighteenth to mid-nineteenth centuries, the medical profession continued to employ the conventional methods of the period. Similar to Greek culture, the physicians of the time saw disease as reflecting imbalances in the four humors of the body—namely, blood, phlegm, yellow bile, and black bile (Estes, 1985). In addition, the imbalances were referred to as excesses or deficits of heat and cold or moisture and dryness. As remedies, doctors used energetic, aggressive ways to fight disease with little awareness of the harmful effects of their treatments (Stewart, 1990). Barbaric and unscientific techniques, including bleeding and purging patients, became preferred methods that not infrequently caused death (Weil, 1983). The use of cathartics and emetics, believed to rid the body of the noxious materials thought to cause disease, also prevailed, and physicians prescribed a wide range of drugs to treat each symptom rather than the illness as a whole (Estes, 1985). Thus, this period was called the Age of Heroic Medicine.

Such practices outraged the public and led to the establishment of the Popular Movement in the United States, which concentrated on improving the quality of life mainly through diet and exercise. Formed in reaction to the abysmal state of medical practices, its proponents touted the slogan " every man, his own doctor" which represented a battlecry for responsibility and self-determination in health care (Weil, 1983, p. 21).

On the heels of this philosophy, the nineteenth century popularized the *cold-water cure*, first introduced into the United States in the early 1800s. According to Cayeleff (1988), hydrotherapy offered flexible, hygienic principles in lieu of drug-based therapeutics, with moderate regimens ensuring purification and absolution. It also promoted the concept of *home self-doctoring*, awakening the patient's innate healing powers as well as arousing hope and possibility for a cure (p. 83). Women found hydrotherapy especially attractive because its proponents viewed physiological processes such as childbirth and menopause as natural phenomena rather than illnesses.

Because the water cures were offered within institutional-like settings, they provided relief away from home chores and daily routines. Susan B. Anthony, the prominent feminist, found hydrotherapy invigorating, challenging, and absorbing and described her experience as follows:

> First thing in the morning dripping sheet pack at 10 o'clock for 45 minutes. . . .take a shower followed by a sitz bath with a pail of water at 75 degrees poured over the shoulders after which a dry sheet, then brisk exercises. At 4 P.M., the program repeated, and then again at 9 P.M. My day is so cut up with four baths, four dressings and undressings, four exercisings, one drive and three eatings, that I do not have time to put two thoughts together. (Cayeleff, 1988, p. 93)

Hydrotherapy continues today in the form of whirlpool baths, saunas, and home jacuzzis. As suggested by its more ancient roots, such as the Roman baths and the Indian sweat lodges, the results produce comfort, hygiene, and relaxation.

With the launching of modern nursing in the late 1800s, Florence Nightingale brought respectability to the profession and redefined health worldwide. Against the wishes of her parents, she studied with the deaconesses at Kaiserworth, in Germany, and succeeded later in changing nursing's image through education and the cultivation of more humanistic values. In defining the two major categories of health nursing and sick nursing, she cited caring for the sick and helping people to stay healthy as primary goals (Doheny, Cook, & Stopper, 1982).

In her view, every woman had the potential for assuming the role of the nurse. The preface to her *Notes on Nursing* (1859) pointed to the need for educating nurses in the care of the sick:

> . . .if [only] every woman would think how to be a nurse. I do not pretend to teach her how, I ask her to teach herself, and for this purpose I venture to give her some hints. (p. 1)

Nightingale's approach to healing involved "fresh air, medications, quiet, mobility, piped hot water, a call bell system for patients, cleanliness, and comfort" (Doheny, Cook, & Stopper, 1982, p. 57). She cited the first canon of nursing as keeping "the air the patient breathes as pure as the external air without chilling him" (Nightingale, 1859, p. 8), and she maintained that the five essential points in securing the health of a house included pure air and water, efficient drainage, cleanliness, and light. Another need, related to diet, varied according to the sick person's capacity to tolerate food.

Among Nightingale's reforms was the call for a change in surroundings, urging patients to pursue such activities as painting, coloring, music, working with flowers and plants, and spending time with pets and children to aid recovery (Watson, 1999). In addition, she discussed the psychological as well as the physical aspects of illness, suggesting that a wholeness existed that should not be divided into parts. "The sick suffer to excess from mental as well as bodily pain," Nightingale observed, and "humor and colorful surroundings can help the patient to overcome feelings of distress" (p. 84).

As nursing and medicine moved into the twentieth century, it was apparent that the scientific, reductionistic approach overshadowed most other healing practices in the Western world. Trained to diagnose clinical patterns of disease, physicians applied their knowledge in a broad variety of settings. The discovery of drugs and vaccines helped conquer communicable diseases, and more radical surgical procedures and technology gave new hope for extending human life. Discoveries such as vitamins, hormones, and antibiotics became widely used in preventing or treating a variety of conditions (Weil, 1983; Stewart, 1990). Although health care improved, it became apparent that the healing power of nature and more holistic views of health were drifting further into the background (Porter, 1997).

During the 1970s, a holistic health movement was resurrected in reaction to the growing dissatisfaction with the traditional medical establishment's major approaches to healing, namely surgery and drugs. Although effective for acute conditions that required timely and aggressive interventions, these methods proved to be far less appropriate for chronic illnesses that were developing and progressing over time. Identified as alternative therapies, holistic treatments did not convey the notion of choosing one over the other. With the arrival of the twenty-first century, health care consumers began to expand their knowledge and scope of interests, exploring a variety of approaches within an emerging integrated health care model.

SUMMARY

Thousands of years ago, the healer's focus on the mind, body, and spirit of the individual as a complete entity was the rule and not the exception. Even with their ritualistic practices and beliefs in the supernatural, societies of yesteryear approached healing from a holistic perspective. Nowhere was this more evident than in the ancient healing temples of Greece, in the philosophy of the Father of Medicine, and in the theories regarding the prevention and environmental influences espoused by the founder of modern nursing. Although nursing has undergone a marked shift in role over the centuries—beginning with the medicine woman of antiquity and leading up to modern, integrated approaches to health care—nursing's most singular constant endures: *it is ability of the nurse to care and heal.*

DISCUSSION GUIDE

1. Explore the history of healing practices, and explain why it has relevance and/or applicability to modern health care.
2. Identify the similarities and differences in the healing practices of four ancient cultures.
3. Discuss the impact of women healers throughout the ages.

4. Discuss the advent of scientific medicine and how its approaches to healing affected the practice of nursing in both positive and negative ways.
5. Describe Florence Nightingale's views and how they apply to nursing in the twenty-first century.

REFERENCES

Abrahamsen, V. (1997). The goddess and healing: Nursing's heritage from antiquity. *Journal of Holistic Nursing*, 15 (1), 9–24.

Achterberg, J. (1991). *Woman as healer: A panoramic survey of women from prehistoric times to the present.* Boston: Shambala.

Beinfield, H., & Korngold, L. (1991). *Between heaven and earth: A guide to Chinese medicine.* New York: Ballantine.

Cayeleff, S. E. (1988). Gender, ideology and the water cure movement. In N. Gevitz (Ed.), *Other healers: Unorthodox medicine in America* (pp. 82–98). Baltimore: Johns Hopkins.

Doheny, M., Cook, C., & Stopper, M. (1982). *The discipline of nursing: An introduction.* Bowie, MD: Brady.

Dolan, J., Fitzpatrick, M. L., & Hermann, E. K. (1983). *Nursing in society: A historical perspective* (15th ed.). Philadelphia: Saunders.

Ehenreich, B., & English, D. (1973). *Witches, midwives and nurses: A history of women healers.* New York: Feminist Press.

Estes, J. W. (1985). George Washington and the doctors: Treating America's first superhero. *Medical Heritage*, 1 (1), 12–13.

Ghalioungui, P. (1963). *Magic and medical science in ancient Egypt.* London: Hodder and Stoughton.

Keegan, L. (1994). *The nurse as healer.* Albany, NY: Delmar.

Kelly, L. Y., & Joel, L. A. (1995). *Dimensions of professional nursing* (7th ed.). New York: McGraw-Hill.

Krieger, D. (1981). *Foundations for holistic health nursing practices: The renaissance nurse.* Philadelphia: Lippincott.

Lefkowitz, M. R., & Fant, M. B. (1982). *Women's life in Greece and Rome.* Baltimore: Johns Hopkins.

Lindemans, M. F. (2000). *The coming of medicine.* Encyclopedia Mythica. http://www.pantheon.org/

Masson, M. (1985). *A pictorial history of nursing.* Twickenham, Middlesex, UK: Hamlyn.

Nightingale, F. (1859). *Notes on nursing: What it is and what it is not.* London: Harrison.

Porter, R. (1997). *The greatest benefit to mankind: A medical history of humanity.* New York: Norton.

Reis, P. (1991). *Through the goddess: A woman's way of healing.* New York: Continuum.

Scarborough, J. (1969). *Roman medicine: Aspects of Greek and Roman life.* Ithaca, NY: Cornell University Press.

Stewart, G. (1990). *Great mysteries: Alternative healing: Opposing viewpoints.* San Diego: Greenhaven.

Watson, J. (1999). *Postmodern nursing and beyond.* New York: Churchill Livingstone.

Weil, A. (1983). *Health and healing: Understanding conventional and alternative medicine.* Boston: Houghton Mifflin.

CHAPTER 2

THE HEALERS: WHO THEY ARE AND HOW THEY HEAL

Maintaining order rather than correcting disorder is the ultimate principle of wisdom. To cure disease after it has appeared is like digging a well when one already feels thirsty, or forging weapons after the war has already begun.

H. Beinfield & E. Korngold, *Between Heaven and Earth*

Nurses, physicians, and other professionals may perceive themselves as healers, but their approaches, philosophically and practically, may differ among practitioners. Before embarking on their journey into the healing realm, certain factors must be kept in mind. Of primary importance is a recognition of their attitudes toward the healing process, including the expected level of healer and patient involvement, which may depend to a large extent not only on the individual but also on the health care environment. Another factor relates to how healers perceive themselves and their motivation in pursuing particular healing practices.

Many people believe that the drive toward self-healing is one of the most basic human characteristics, ascribing it particularly to the helping professions (Brennan, 1993; Small, 1990). Although this view is not always seen in a positive light, the misperception still exists that individuals must be free from problems to be effective healers. Jung (1951) reminds us that in light of the professional's vulnerability, wholeness rather than "clean hands perfection" represents a core virtue of the healing process. His observation has relevance for nurses because they have been taught to value flawlessness in their practice. Yet, perfection can pose stumbling blocks in helping patients heal, because it may be an unrealistic goal.

Although some authorities argue that such activities as physical treatments or varied techniques are the major components of the healing process, others purport that healers do not really heal but act as a mirror to help patients see themselves (Andrews, 1989). According to Brennan (1993), the gift of healing rests with everyone and the process becomes developmental in nature requiring dedication, love, truthfulness, and faith. Growth, tests, and adversity also enable healers to find direction. Furthermore, healers must realize that a deeper meaning occurs within each person's experience of illness and that even death does not imply failure to heal (Brennan, 1987).

Nurses as wounded healers initially need to identify their fundamental beliefs about healing modalities along with the more significant aspect of engendering self-awareness. To effect positive outcomes in their patients, they require knowledge and understanding of the healing process as well as the various techniques employed. Carlson & Shield (1989) describe the nature of the healing relationship:

> From the joining of the hearts and minds comes the realization that we are indeed one in our suffering. In the presence of this relationship, both healer and client explore the depth of their experiences and resources. It is through this unity that both parties can indeed be healed. (p. 83)

THEORETICAL APPROACHES TO HEALING

The Reductionistic Perspective

The interrelatedness of the concepts "curing" and "healing" sheds some light on why certain practices generate more effective patient outcomes. To illuminate the dialogue, we may acquire more helpful insights through an analysis of reductionism and holism. As a theoretical approach commonly associated with the Western model of medicine, reductionism is applied when the health practitioner perceives the human body or disease entity in terms of its smallest possible parts or forms. Such a view implies "causality," assuming that a new awareness of the health problem can be elicited and a definitive answer identified.

Reductionistic methods aim toward achieving a cure, based on the belief that by applying scientific principles, the cause of illness will be determined largely through analyzing anatomical structures or body chemistry. Unfortunately, the cause of a particular illness may not always be that precise. There must be a realization that even when cure is possible, it tends to provide a more temporary and palliative effect and does not necessarily address the underlying causes of the illness (Upledger, 1989).

In certain mental illnesses, for example, the cause appears to be at the cellular level, reflected by excesses or depletion of neurotransmitters in the brain that can affect emotions and behavior. Not all these conditions, however, respond well to treatment with medication. Although a depressed individual may initially have a favorable reaction to a drug that alters the neurotransmitter levels in the brain, recovery from the depression may be short-lived. Such an outcome seems to suggest that the symptoms could be due to more than merely a chemical imbalance or that the body-mind adapts to the medication rendering it ineffective.

Another example may occur in opiate addiction—also manifested by neurotransmitter imbalances—when we observe that the sole use of methadone treatment to address the physiological symptoms rarely resolves the problem. By applying reductionism, the treatment of disease has been perceived primarily as symptom control, which often reflects an inadequate approach to healing the affected person. Although reductionistic methods are usually more effective in treating acute illnesses, they often foster a high potential for iatrogenic disease or harmful side effects. To illustrate, some medications have untoward effects, but the benefit must outweigh the risk of taking them.

Traditionally, health care professionals who practice reductionistically may unwittingly demonstrate a paternalistic attitude that can deter patients from assuming more responsibility for the results of their treatment as well as for their own general health. Since this approach uses technologies largely derived from scientific methods, treatments depend on information interpreted by the prescribing practitioner and the patient, who until recent years, raised few questions or concerns. This "do as I say" model becomes counterproductive particularly if the healer is not a positive role model for a healthy lifestyle: An obese or visibly overstressed caregiver will not be taken seriously by the patient.

Finally, since reductionists view illness as having prescribed patterns, this approach can lead to a lack of individualized treatment for patients who do not conform to a certain mold and respond to preordained protocols—a situation more prevalent than acknowledged. Common examples include fatigue and muscle aches that cannot be attributed to a particular physical cause as reflected in laboratory tests. Hence, a visit to the physician's office may fail to provide the positive outcome for a particular health problem that cannot be measured using reductionistic tools.

When reductionistic healers are unable to eradicate disease, they encounter a dilemma and may convey to the patient that nothing further can be done. Regrettably, such cases carry the sting of "treatment failures" by Western medical standards and, even when harbored unconsciously, hopeless attitudes have a detrimental effect on the individual's will to be healed. Simonton (1984), a physician, explains his view of the need to separate the healer from the doctor as follows:

> The physician is trained in the prevailing beliefs of the medical profession. If the patient can view those beliefs as simply one person's beliefs, rather than being overwhelmed by the doctor's authority and taking those beliefs as truth, he can be more aware of the type of care he is receiving. This becomes very important in helping a person deal with a physician who believes there is no chance for cure or even any significant chance for improvement. (p. 51)

The Holistic Perspective

In contrast to the practice of reductionism, holism has assumed an entirely different approach within the healing domain. Function-oriented, it emphasizes that the whole is greater than the sum of its parts and that human beings and the environment are energy systems which incorporate dynamic forces contributing to ever-changing rather than fixed diagnoses. Certain principles stress the interrelatedness of organ systems and the mind-body as a single entity.

Employing the term "body-mind," Achterberg & Lawlis (1980) perceive the individual as the total collection of receptive and reactive units capable of responding to one another and the environment. Consequently, any disturbance in one part of the system affects the entire organism: the body, mind, and spirit. Philosophically, holism focuses on the identification, treatment, and balancing of patterns of disharmony and the awakening of innate health. From this perspective, symptoms of illness can be seen as "signals for attention or ways of making us aware that our needs are not being met" (Rossman, 1989, p. 79). Ascribing to this point of view helps the person look beyond symptomatology in the effort to become healed.

Holistic treatment incorporates a melange of beliefs, techniques, and pharmacological therapies, not necessarily united in a common system. When its proponents reentered the health care scene in the 1970s, they introduced unconventional methods (by Western standards) such as the use of herbs, massage, acupuncture, natural medications, and concoctions to the exclusion of allopathic remedies. Most holistic practitioners consider healing to be a natural process within individuals that extends beyond the results that follow intervention. By using the principle of a therapeutic alliance, a "do as I do" approach, they focus on the person rather than the disease.

Since some illnesses have similar presentations, they realize that individuals do not necessarily respond in the same manner to a particular course of treatment. Prevention, being wellness-based, becomes a key element, and thus some holistic techniques seem infinitely better-suited to helping people with chronic illnesses. While iatrogenic side effects may occur, such as adverse drug interactions from some herbal preparations, the risk appears to be much lower than when employing reductionistic methods.

In more recent times, feminist perceptions about the holistic nature of nursing have resurrected some older methods of care, including various massage techniques and aromatherapy that had been practiced for thousands of years (Buckle, 1997). Within nurse-patient interactions, a sharing of beliefs and concerns about life and health evolves, producing an open interchange that encourages decision making by the affected person in a therapeutic climate. Through patient teaching and role modeling of healthy behaviors, nurses help expedite the healing process. Whorton (1988) reproduces an interesting quote from a Mr. Dooley, an obscure figure in the early twentieth century, who verifies what every nurse knows: "If the Christyan Scientists had some science and the doctors more Christyanity, it wudden't make anny dif-f'rence which ye call in—if ye had a good nurse" (p. 52).

Unquestionably, the manner in which healers approach relationships depends markedly on their theoretical orientation and attitudes. Both reductionistic and holistic practitioners may be short-sighted, however, if they favor extremes of one method to the exclusion of others. An integrative approach is by far the best in fostering healing and increasing patient satisfaction with treatment outcomes, even when cure seems unlikely. In modern health care, the preventive pattern has assumed increasing prominence because patients are seeking alternative or complementary therapies when traditional Western medical approaches fail to elicit the expected results.

HEALING APPROACHES AND OUTCOMES

Experts such as Andrew Weil (1983) and others have examined the various types of healing approaches necessary for acquiring an understanding of the wounded healer. Practitioners use different modalities ranging on a continuum from the most physical to the spiritual or ethereal.

Healing the Physical Body

Methods employed to heal the physical body closely follow the reductionistic philosophy. Although certain medications or surgical techniques have an impact on healing, the level of patient participation may seem to remain fairly passive or even detached. Whereas psychological and spiritual factors such as the will to live and belief in the effectiveness of the treatment generally enter into the healing process, the focus of the healer's involvement remains on curing the physical wound.

Who then are these practitioners and how do they perform? Within this group predominantly falls the allopathic physician. The term allopathic was coined by a German doctor named Hahnemann. This homeopathic scientist, who practiced in the early twentieth century, is credited to be the first person to describe allopathy as a medical treatment based on the law of contraries. The term "allopathic," a combination of the Greek words *allo* and *pathos*, means "other than disease" because the drugs prescribed for a particular health problem have no logical relationship to symptoms (Weil, 1983). Unlike homeopathy, which uses drugs or treatments to support the symptoms or increase their intensity to stimulate the body's natural defense against the illness, allopathy employs antagonists such as specific antihypertensive and antipyretic medications to counteract the symptoms and thereby eliminate them. Ironically, Hahnemann became the founder of modern-day homeopathy after becoming disillusioned with the allopathic practices of his day.

By virtue of their education, the majority of physicians can be classified as allopaths. Other types of doctors, such as osteopaths (D.O.), also treat patients and largely duplicate the role and functions of M.D.s, but they represent a separate genre (Gevitz, 1988). Founded by Andrew Taylor Still, in the early nineteenth century, the practice of osteopathy focuses on bone treatment. In his practice, Taylor Still eliminated the use of drugs and tried to promote healing by "manipulating bones to allow free circulation of blood and balanced functioning of nerves" (Weil, 1983, p. 125). He pointed out that malfunction of joints "stopped the flow of blood at that point and so reduced the ability to produce chemicals to fight illness" (Camp, 1973 p. 137).

The cardinal principle underlying modern osteopathy is that when a restoration of the blood circulation occurs, the body can deal with disease in its own way (Camp, 1973). Osteopaths tend to harbor a somewhat more holistic philosophy than other allopaths, believing that in studying health and disease, no single part of the body can be considered autonomous. They also hold that health and treatment of disease can be accomplished only through the study of the whole person in relation to the internal and external environments (Osteopathy Canada, 1998).

Most allopathic, homeopathic, and modern osteopathic medical treatments involve the dispensing of drugs. Patients participate in the healing process according to the physician's instructions and must be convinced that the medication will work. The material nature of allopathic practices and healing methods emanates from an analysis of symptoms, laboratory tests, and the individual's medical history that form the basis for diagnosis and treatment. In their perception of health as the absence of disease, allopaths give credence to no particular idea or theory about the illness or to any general view of treatment. The result has been a proliferation of cumbersome data that identify specific physical causes of disease and suggest particular treatments to cure, remove, or eliminate them (Weil, 1983). Unfortunately, diagnosis and treatment can become difficult when certain health problems do not follow the descriptions outlined in medical sources.

In their reliance on medications, homeopaths base their treatment on administering a drug resembling the disease itself. In this way, the body mobilizes itself against the illness and an immediate worsening of symptoms appears, similar to the rallying of the immune system followed by a cure (Zand, Spreen, & LaValle, 1999). For example, *allium*, a homeopathic remedy derived from the red onion used to cure colds, produces a burning nasal discharge and watering eyes, not unlike symptoms caused by slicing an onion. Another treatment, the *eyebright* plant, is fancied by some to cure eye afflictions because its flowers resemble an eye (Camp, 1973; Aesoph, 2000).

In spite of the premise "like cures like" that originally stemmed from the outward resemblance of the symptom or organ to the plant represented, Hahnemann's theory asserts that the capacity of the plant to heal can be attributed more to an ability to generate similar symptoms of the disease but only in modified form (Camp, 1973). Perhaps one of the most famous substances to illustrate this point is Peruvian bark, which *induces* fever when administered to afebrile individuals. It also has use as an antidote for malaria, especially in *reducing* fever.

Within the healing spectrum, homeopathy extends beyond allopathic medicine, since it also includes spiritual beliefs. Hahnemann has observed that the spiritual essence of the drug creates a greater impact than its physical properties and therefore is more important than the material reality.

Edward Bach (1931) has shown the relationship between spirituality and drug treatment by introducing flower essences, remedies prepared only with water, sunlight, and certain types of flowers or plants, with a total of 38. Their action, he explains, raises the individual's vibrations and opens up the channels to receive spiritual energy as well as to eradicate the cause of harm (Scheffer, 1988). Bach views the ills of the heart and the spirit as the focus of the practitioner's intention and self-knowledge or as the gateway to the healer's success (Bach & Wheeler, 1997; Scheffer, 1988). Applying his technique requires the patient to determine what remedy to ingest and for how long by reviewing all the flower essences and their characteristics. Usually four or five are selected, diluted in water, and taken about four times a day. Because no side effects are anticipated, the essences may be taken with all other types of medications.

In situations of personal crisis, an example of a specific formula that might be chosen could include a combination of such essences as the Star of Bethlehem for sudden shock, Sweet Chestnut for severe mental anguish, Elm for being overwhelmed by unexpected responsibility, and Rock Rose for terror. The use of flower essences has proved to be effective in that the vibrations within them interact with the subtle energy of the patient and heal and harmonize at the spiritual, mental, and emotional levels (Original Bach Flower Essences, 1999). These remedies generally may be self-prescribed and purchased over the counter at many health food stores.

Mind and Faith Healing

The expression "mind and faith healing" has a familiar ring to most of us with its practitioners abounding. Theoretically, it cannot be perceived within the material realm, since the approach requires the individual to believe that healing will occur. As such, mind-mediated healing takes place because of the confidence in the healer or the healing method (Stewart, 1990). Well known to many believers is the practice of Christian Science, whose founder Mary Baker Eddy endured a precarious state of health from infancy. Most predominant among her symptoms were seizures that seemed to be related to her emotional state, and often precipitated by bouts of anger (Dakin, 1968).

Severely injured at the age of 45, after slipping on a patch of ice, Eddy suffered a concussion and spinal dislocation (Pickering, 1974). During her convalescence, while perusing a Bible passage recounting Christ's cure of a man with palsy, she claimed a sudden realization of how to heal herself and attained complete recovery. From this "awakening," she concluded that disease, pain, injury, and death were illusions due to the individual's mistaken thoughts considered to be real and given the power to influence health (Daken, 1968; Weil, 1983).

As its basic premise, Christian Science ideology purports that healing energy can be retrieved from a benevolent force ruling the universe through a properly attuned mind. Its followers turn scrupulously to prayer, attempting to focus on the goodness of the spirit and directing its infinite energy to promote healing (Weil, 1983). Christian Scientists believe that because their ailments are illusory in nature, the symptoms will disappear by practicing their faith.

Faith healing practices are ubiquitous with many of the approaches differing markedly from Christian Scientists. These healers often appear in fundamentalist sects of Christianity and use the Bible and the miracles of Jesus Christ as a model for their work. Most of them espouse the dogma that human beings endure pain, suffering, disease, and death because they are tainted by original sin, and they attribute failure to heal as the punishment for sins or simply as God's will (Weil, 1983).

These practitioners often display several commonalities with some professing to be ministers, although lacking formal theological training or academic degrees. Oral Roberts, an internationally known healer, who achieved a modicum of respectability, contends that he has healed a variety of disorders including cancer, tuberculosis, and paralysis (Flammonde, 1999). The son of a Pentecostal preacher, supposedly cured of tuberculosis at the age of sixteen by a faith healer, Roberts claims to have made the blind see, to have raised the dead, and to have actually met a "900 foot tall Christ!" (Flammonde, 1999, p. 61).

Earlier in the twentieth century, Aimee Semple McPherson became one of the most famous faith healers. Born to the daughter of a Salvation Army worker and a Pentecostal minister, she claimed to have had a near-death experience at the age of 23. She initiated a traveling ministry across the United States and Canada, attracting huge audiences as she preached her gospel. Garbed in a white flowing gown, she presided over a white temple in California, a Mecca for those seeking to be healed. Radio broadcasts increased her popularity.

As with many other faith healers, McPherson's life generated scandal when "kidnapped" under highly suspicious circumstances. After disappearing while clad only in a swimsuit, she reappeared 13 days later fully clothed after supposedly escaping from her captors. At the time, her shoes showed no indication of a 13-hour hike through the desert, nor could the house be found where she claimed to have been held captive. Although indicted for perjury regarding the episode, the charges were eventually dropped (Blumhoffer, 1993; Epstein, 1993). Until her death from a barbiturate overdose in 1944, she continued to draw large crowds to her temple services.

Other types of faith healing include pilgrimages to sacred places or the touching of saints' relics. A familiar site is the well-known shrine at Lourdes, France, where St. Bernadette proclaimed to have visions of the Virgin Mary in the 1800s. During one of these apparitions, a spring of flowing water emerged from the rocks in a grotto. Ever since this happening, the immersion of an infirm or a handicapped person in the spring has been associated with many miraculous cures recognized by the Catholic Church (Stewart, 1990). In one case, a patient was reported to have tuberculosis of the lung and bone, and after immersing himself in the waters at the shrine, he recovered with only a slight scar over one bone as a reminder of his illness (Bengtsson, 1995). Visitors to Lourdes may collect water from the spring to help with any petitions for healing that may arise in the future.

The Western Wall in Jerusalem, often referred to as the Wailing Wall, is also a revered site. The Wall is what remains of a massive porch that once surrounded the Temple, the holiest place of prayer for the Jewish people, which was built by Herod the Great and destroyed by the Romans in 70 A.D. At the Wall, people often insert a written prayer on a small piece of paper into one of the many cracks, believing that their supplications will be answered.

It is not unusual that relics associated with a saint or martyr often become highly venerated objects. Some people believe that by possessing or touching a relic they will be healed or granted special favors by the saint. A well-known example has been the relics of the French Carmelite nun St. Thérèse of Lisieux, who was elevated to sainthood after her death at the age of 24 from tuberculosis. Not until her autobiography *The Story of a Soul* was published in 1898 did the extraordinary gifts of the "Little Flower" become known (Beevers, 1989). The work of St. Thérèse revealed such a high level of spirituality that she merited the title Doctor of the Church. She was only the third woman in the history of Catholicism to receive this honor, bestowed for outstanding holiness and sanctity. In the spring of 2000, her relic bones and other remains were transported to the United States for people to view as part of a worldwide movement to publicize her sanctity and restore interest in the Catholic faith.

A commentary on faith healing would be incomplete without mentioning the fraudulent activity of "practitioners" who prey on the vulnerabilities of the sick and needy. Nowhere is this type of person more aptly demonstrated than in Sinclair Lewis' riveting novel *Elmer Gantry*, published in 1927. Probably the greatest satirist of his era, Lewis depicted Gantry as the scandalous and charismatic salesman who became an evangelical revivalist and performed "miracles" in his Bible Belt meetings. Unfortunately, such charlatans continue to exist in real life and often succeed in achieving their goals of fame and fortune.

Psychic Healing

One of the most esoteric and controversial modalities falls under the rubric of psychic healing. Originating in ancient times with the shamans, it sprang from the notion of healing emanating from a spiritual experience (Stewart, 1990). In contemporary life, many psychic healers attune themselves to the spiritual world to guide and direct the energy required for healing. This activity can be accomplished through the intercession of "spirit helpers," human, animal, or plant entities that can be called upon at will for guidance or through the process of channeling between the spiritual and physical worlds for the healing energies of the universe.

During the 1950s and 1960s, José Arigo achieved notable visibility as a psychic healer in Brazil. Although not a medical doctor, he amazed onlookers who observed him diagnosing disease and surgically removing diseased tissue or malignant growths (Stewart, 1990). Assuming a trancelike appearance, he employed several spirit guides, including a German physician who had died in World War I, a year before Arigo's birth. During the trances, he spoke German, a language he had never studied. People claimed to have witnessed his surgeries being performed with a rusty knife, used repeatedly on a number of unanesthetized patients in relatively bloodless operations without subsequent infection. After decades of psychic healing, Arigo was killed in a motor vehicle accident in 1971.

In the early seventies, thousands of colleagues, disciples, and beneficiaries honored Harry Edwards, a psychic healer, in London's Royal Albert Hall on the occasion of his eightieth birthday (Flammonde, 1999). Known as the world's greatest healer, it was estimated that 35 percent of his patients had been cured. He believed that all healing had a "divine source carried out by God's ministers in spirit or healing intelligences" (p. 149).

Edwards derived his skill from both "hands on" healing and "absent healing," or healing from a distance. In one case, a woman contacted him about her husband who had been diagnosed with advanced liver cancer. The day after Edwards focused on the man's healing, the patient was purportedly cured without knowing the source of his dramatic recovery. Although skepticism continues regarding psychic healing, it remains the subject of considerable research and interest around the world.

Energy Healing

In contrast to other types of practitioners, energy healers appear at the opposite end of the continuum. They believe that matter consists of energy, with illness occurring as an imbalance in the human energy field produced by various internal or external causes. Healing of this nature requires rebalancing the energy field and identifying the causes and meanings of illness to prevent recurrence. These healers base their practice on the premise that no real separation exists between human beings and the environment. Rather, the entire universe represents a dynamic whole composed of a web of inseparable patterns, with the healer and patient engaged in a relationship that focuses on the factors to be addressed for healing to take place (Brennan, 1987).

Energy healing involves noncontact modalities such as Therapeutic Touch (TT), which emerged in the early 1970s from the work of Dolores Krieger, a nurse, and Dora Kunz, a healer claiming to be clairvoyant from birth. Kunz perceived the aura, or energy fields, that surrounded individuals and often helped medical practitioners to diagnose and treat illness by visualizing imbalances in a person's auric field.

Krieger acquired the skill of "laying on of hands" from Kunz, followed by several years of formulating her TT theory and practice. She introduced this healing modality at New York University Hospital, where she has taught nurses how to incorporate it into their practice. During the process, practitioners center themselves and use the natural sensitivity of the hands to assess the patterns of energy flow throughout the patient's body and to release blockages in the energy field.

Healers employing Krieger's approach apply energy to assist individuals in repatterning their own energies (Krieger, 1979; Quinn, 1999). This transfer of energy "boosts" the patient's recuperative system and tends to accelerate the healing process (Krieger, 1979). Studies on Therapeutic Touch have shown it to be effective for a variety of conditions, such as reducing anxiety and pain management (Heidt, 1981; Apostle-Mitchell & MacDonald, 1997). Nurse healers have continued to practice this modality, as demonstrated by Madrid (1994) in her care of the dying.

As another energy healing method formulated by nurses, Healing Touch (HT) involves both contact and noncontact. With its roots in TT and the art of caring, HT comes from the heart of the healer who transmits it to the person receiving help (Mentgen, 1996). Healing Touch includes TT techniques such as centering and assessing the energy field along with contact techniques such as full-body hands-on healing. More specifically, it supports what is called an endogenous healing process, which suggests that only patients can heal themselves.

Developed by Dorothy Hover-Kramer, Janet Mentgen, and Sharon Scandrett-Hibdon (1996), HT consists of six elements: awareness, appraisal, choosing, acceptance, alignment, and outcome. As patients become *aware* of cues within the internal and external environments, they perceive disturbances and identify potential health problems. Next, an *appraisal* period occurs in which they explore and evaluate what the newly acquired awareness has brought to their consciousness and to the meanings and relationships of past and present health patterns. *Choosing* refers to how clients respond to their disharmony, whether it be a learning tool or a phenomena to be avoided.

During the process, *acceptance* allows healing energy to flow more freely, or conversely, in nonacceptance the individual fails to deal with his or her circumstance. With the achieving of *alignment*, there follows an integration of the internal and external actions that support movement toward harmony, shifting the energy toward the goal of healing (p. 21). Finally, the *endpoint*, or *outcome*, generates a sense of being harmonious and experiencing a sense of wholeness (p. 21). As a philosophical foundation, the endogenous healing process represents another contribution to the development of the nurse as wounded healer.

Among energy healers has evolved the method known as AMMA Therapy, a form of therapeutic body work based on Traditional Chinese Medicine (TCM). Introduced in the United States by Tina Sohn in the 1970s, this approach energizes the system through various manipulations of the physical body, appropriate diet, and exercise. By emphasizing "my hands are my eyes and ears," Sohn illustrates the nature and importance of the healing touch (Sohn & Sohn, 1996).

Born into a Korean family with a long healing tradition, she received her training beginning in childhood, primarily in therapeutic body work. At age 12, she suffered a great emotional loss from the deaths of her father and brother and fell into a coma that lasted 30 days. On awakening, Sohn became extremely sensitive to the pain and illness of others and developed the capacity to detect an ailment that she knew how to heal. Through the use of touch, she effected the healing process with the application of AMMA Therapy.

The value of using this approach has been demonstrated in addressing certain imbalances. Anneke Young (1993), a Dutch nurse, has used body work, herbs, and diet modification to enhance immune system response, promote a greater sense of well-being, reduce pain, and improve the level of functioning in such conditions as chronic fatigue syndrome. AMMA Therapy is rapidly becoming an exciting new healing modality for nurses and other health professionals.

The ancient healing art Reiki, which means "universal energy," also represents a popular method, particularly useful for stress reduction and relaxation and involves the laying on of hands (Rand, 1998). Unlike TT, which excludes body contact or AMMA Therapy that may involve intense physical involvement, Reiki operates through touch but without physical manipulation, and functions on the principle that both practitioner and patient have a strong need to be healed.

During the treatment, the Rei, or God-conscious part of the energy, assesses where blocks occur in the individual and then directs the healing energy to the blocked area closest to the hands (Rand, 1998, p. 5). Not perceived as a religion, Reiki assumes a Higher Power and Higher Consciousness, manifested through the life force Ki. The technique also deals with negative thought patterns and feelings that curtail the natural flow of energy, thereby releasing and balancing the pathways (Rand, 1998).

Often used interchangeably, the terms "energy healing" and "spiritual healing" encompass both human and universal energy fields. Although spirituality tends to be confused with religiosity or a strong adherence to organized religion, a clearer definition can be found in the word *shen-jing* in Traditional Chinese Medicine. *Shen* originates from the spirit and forms the outward expression of the organism, including the health or physical appearance, along with the focus, lucidity, and intensity of the intellectual and emotional process (Beinfield & Korngold, 1991). On the other hand, *jing* refers to a person's material substance, physical structure, and sensate life.

Shen-jing describes the totality of an individual's experience both tangibly and otherwise, and when the term is applied to the human organism, practitioners understand that manifestations of healing may be either visible or unseen (Beinfield & Korngold, 1991). In addition, major changes must take place in an individual's approach to life in the physical and spiritual realms well before the stages of transformation, transcendence, and healing can take place.

SUMMARY

Persons involved in healing are known to base their practices on a variety of ideologies that reveal several commonalities under the rubric of legitimacy.

Whether the focus rests in the physical or spiritual realm, most healers aim to help patients overcome health imbalances. They need to be knowledgeable as well as circumspect about fraudulent practitioners who continue to exist and prey on the vulnerability of the "true believer" who is seeking a miraculous cure.

Although reductionistic methods still pervade the health care community, creating a growing dissatisfaction, a positive approach in recent decades is the movement toward holistic practice. Nursing exists in the forefront of the shift with the development of new modalities to effect healing outcomes. Most notable are Therapeutic Touch, Healing Touch, AMMA Therapy, and Reiki. Along with the methods used, however, health professionals must recognize the complexity of the healing process and reflect on it in relation to improving themselves and their patients. This process of self-examination is crucial to understanding the wounded healer.

DISCUSSION GUIDE

1. Compare the reductionistic and holistic approaches to healing as they relate to nursing practice. Identify positive and negative features.
2. Among the various healing methods, describe one or two that you personally ascribe to more than others, and indicate why.
3. Contrast the practice of energy healers with their counterparts who employ more traditional methods.
4. Describe the role of the nurse when patients express interest in pursuing faith healing practices.
5. Share your thoughts about healing modalities, such as Bach Flower Essences and pilgrimages to sacred places.

REFERENCES

Achterberg, J., & Lawlis, G. F. (1980). *Bridges of the bodymind: Behavioral approaches to health care.* Champaign, IL: Institute for Personality and Ability Testing.

Aesoph, L. M. (2000). The basics of homeopathy. *Great life: Your guide to health and well-being,* 4, 39–41.

Andrews, L. (1989). Mirroring the life force. In R. Carlson and B. Shield (Eds.), *Healers on healing* (pp. 42–47). New York: Penguin Putnam.

Apostle-Mitchell, M., & MacDonald, G. (1997). An innovative approach to pain management in critical care: Therapeutic touch. CACCN, 8 (3), 19–22.

Bach, E. (1931). *Heal thyself: An explanation of the real cause and cure of disease.* Essex, UK: Daniel.

Bach, E., & Wheeler, F. J. (1997). *The Bach flower remedies.* New Canaan, CT: Keats.

Beevers, J. (Trans.) (1989). *The autobiography of Saint Thérèse of Lisieux : The story of a soul.* New York: Doubleday.

Beinfield, H., & Korngold, L. (1991). *Between heaven and earth: A guide to Chinese medicine.* New York: Ballantine.

Bengtsson, O. (1995). Many doors to healing. In. D. Kunz (Ed.), *Spiritual healing: Doctors examine therapeutic touch and other holistic treatments.* Wheaton, IL: Theosophical Publishing House.

Brennan, B. A. (1987). *Hands of light: A guide to healing through the human energy field.* New York: Bantam.

Brennan, B. A. (1993). *Light emerging: The journey of personal healing.* New York: Bantam.

Blumhofer, E. W. (1993). *Aimee Semple McPherson: Everybody's sister.* Grand Rapids, MI: Eermans.

Buckle, J. (1997). *Clinical aromatherapy in nursing.* London: Arnold.

Camp, J. (1973). *Magic, myth and medicine.* New York: Taplinger.

Carlson, R., & Shield, B. (1989). *Healers on healing.* New York: Penguin Putnam.

Daken, E. (1968). *Mrs. Eddy: The biography of a virginal mind.* Gloucester, MA: Peter Smith.

Epstein, D. M. (1993). *Sister Aimee: The life of Aimee Semple McPherson.* New York: Harcourt Brace Jovanovich.

Flammonde, P. (1999). *The mystic healers: A history of magical medicine.* New York: Scarborough.

Gevitz, N. (Ed.), (1988). *Other healers: Unorthodox medicine in America.* Baltimore: Johns Hopkins.

Heidt, P. (1981). Effect of therapeutic touch on anxiety level of hospitalized patients. *Nursing Research, 30* (1), 32–37.

Hover-Kramer, D., Mentgen, J., & Scandrett-Hibdon, S. (1996). *Healing touch: A resource for health professionals.* Albany, NY: Delmar.

Jung, C. G. (1951). Fundamental questions of psychotherapy. In H. Read, M. Fordham, G. Adler, & W. McGuire (Eds.), *The collected works of C. G. Jung* (p. 116). Princeton, NJ: Princeton University Press.

Krieger, D. (1979). *The Therapeutic Touch: How to use your hands to heal.* Englewood Cliffs, NJ: Prentice-Hall.

Lewis, S. (1927). *Elmer Gantry.* New York: Harcourt, Brace and World.

Madrid, M. (1994). Participating in the dying process. In M. Madrid and E.A.M. Barrett (Eds.), *Rogers' scientific art of nursing practice* (pp. 91–100). New York: NLN.

Mentgen, J. (1996). The clinical practice of Healing Touch. In D. Hover-Kramer, J. Mentgen, & S. Scandrett-Hibdon, *Healing Touch: A resource for health professionals.* (pp. 155–165) Albany, NY: Delmar.

Original Bach® Flower Essences. (1999). *Bach Flower Essences™ for the family.* Oxfordshire, UK: Original Bach® Flower Essences.

Osteopathy Canada. (1998). *Osteopathic Philosophy.* http://osteopathycanada.tripod.com/techniques.html

Pickering, G. (1974). *Creative Malady: Illness in the lives and minds of Charles Darwin, Florence Nightingale, Mary Baker Eddy, Sigmund Freud, Marcel Proust and Elizabeth Barrett Browning.* New York: Oxford.

Quinn, J. (1999). Transpersonal caring and healing. In B. Montgomery-Dossey, L. Keegan, & C. E. Guzzetta (Eds.), Holistic nursing: A handbook for practice (pp. 37–48). Gaithersberg, MD: Aspen.

Rand, W. L. (1998). Reiki: The healing touch: First and second degree manual. Southfield, MI: Vision.

Rossman, M. (1989). Illness as an opportunity for healing. In R. Carlson and B. Shield (Eds.), Healers on healing. (pp. 78–81). New York: Penguin Putnam.

Scheffer, M. (1988). Bach Flower Therapy: Theory and practice. Rochester, VT: Healing Arts.

Simonton, S. M. (1984). The healing family: The Simonton approach for families facing illness. New York: Bantam.

Small, J. (1990). Therapists of the future: Transformers: Personal transformation: The way through. Marina del Ray, CA: DeVorss.

Sohn, T., & Sohn, R. (1996). AMMA therapy: A complete textbook of Oriental bodywork and medical principles. Rochester, VT: Healing Arts.

Stewart, G. (1990). Great mysteries: Alternative healing: Opposing viewpoints. San Diego: Greenhaven.

Upledger, J. (1989). Self-discovery and self-healing. In R. Carlson and B. Shield (Eds), Healers on healing (pp. 67–72). New York: Penguin Putnam.

Weil, A. (1983). Health and healing: Understanding conventional and alternative medicine. Boston: Houghton Mifflin.

Whorton, J. C. (1988). Patient, heal thyself: Popular health reform movements as unorthodox medicine. In N. Gevitz (Ed.), Other healers: Unorthodox medicine in America (pp. 52–81). Baltimore: Johns Hopkins.

Young A. (1993). AMMA therapy: A holistic approach to chronic fatigue. Journal of Holistic Nursing, 11 (2), 172–182.

Zand, J., Spreen, A., & LaValle, J. (1999). Smart medicine for healthier living: A practical A–Z reference to natural and conventional treatment for adults. Garden City Park, NY: Avery.

CHAPTER 3

THE WOUNDED HEALER:
THEORETICAL PERSPECTIVES

In the end, only the wounded physician heals and even he, in the last analysis, cannot heal beyond the extent to which he has healed himself.

L. van der Post, *Jung and the Story of our Time*

Nurses have long understood the meaning of "the healer archetype," or an individual who emphasizes the feeling dimension within therapeutic relationships. As a guiding principle, the healer addresses human beings with love and compassion while highly motivated to generate comfort and further wholeness. This caring quality demonstrated in the nurse-patient interaction reflects a mutual valuing with unconditional positive regard (Hover-Kramer, 2000).

The wounded healer extends beyond superficial descriptions often attributed to healers in general, suggesting an in-depth exploration of the true meaning of the healing experience. Its theoretical foundation can be traced to the Greek mythological characters, Apollo, Chiron, Asclepios, and Philoctetes, as well as the ever-present shaman existing throughout the ages in a variety of cultures.

Precursor to Western medical philosophy and its accompanying paternalism, Apollo represented rational enlightenment, objectivity, and intellectualism (Whan, 1987). Unlike the "infected" Chiron, he was a "mortally clean" god, practicing his medical art through catharsis, purification, and sublimation (Whan, 1987). From this standpoint, healers viewed illness objectively, identifying cause and effect and the prescribed treatment. The Apollonion healing approach, however, proved to be defective in its assumption that healers intrinsically had the capability to help patients heal.

The wounded healer archetype is a challenging model to embrace because it acknowledges and transcends personal suffering and a willingness to accept the vulnerability of both practitioner and patient. Within this context, an individual's suffering does not involve becoming totally identified with the pain, but rather cultivates the ability to view it as part of human growth and development.

The legend of Chiron clearly illustrates the meaning of suffering and its relationship to the wounded healer. Derived from the Greek *chirurgia*, the centaur's name meant "working with the hands" (Groesbeck, 1975, p. 126). After accidentally receiving an incurable and painful wound from Herakles' arrow which made him permanently lame, Chiron's fate appeared sealed and he retreated to his cave. Because of his immortality, he could not die from the poison causing the wound, but he moved beyond his anguish to heal others.

By enduring the pain of Prometheus, who had been punished by the gods for stealing fire and giving it to mortal men, Chiron entered Hades, an act which signified transformation, transcendence, and a limit to his suffering (Whan, 1987). Although his wound never healed, he emerged as a wounded healer because of a conscious desire to change his circumstances through sacrifice. In one sense, his story can be viewed as a paradox, since Chiron's suffering remained at the core, yet he transformed his wounding into a positive experience.

Another figure closely associated with the origin of the wounded healer was Asclepios, son of Apollo, the divine physician. After Apollo killed his wife for infidelity, Asclepios was sent to study with Chiron, who taught him about the healing powers of plants, particularly one called Chironion believed to cure snakebites (Early, 1993).

Of interest is that the Asclepios myth revealed the interrelatedness of healing and wounding through the symbol of the caduceus, a staff with a snake encircling it. Interpreted as a renewal of life, the snake typified healing and freedom from illness because of the ability to shed its skin (Meier, 1967). When wrapped around a tree or staff, it represented transcendence, healing, and rebirth (Groesbeck, 1975). In this same light, the caduceus is symbolic of the wounded healer.

Greek literature has provided us with further examples of the wounded healer, most notably in Sophocles' classic work *Philoctetes* (May, 1985). While fighting in the Trojan War, the hero, Philoctetes, armed with the magical bow and arrows of Herakles, was conducting a sacrifice to the gods when bitten by a snake. The bite caused a festering and offensive wound that would not heal. Agamemnon, the commander, was compelled to banish him to the island of Lemnos because of the malodorous infection and the victim's unceasing cries of agony. There, Philoctetes remained in isolation for eight years, using his magic weapons that would unerringly hit any target, including birds for food.

One day, Helenos, a Trojan seer, declared that only by the arrows of Herakles could the Greeks win the city of Troy (Rose, 1960). Dispatched by Agamemnon to the island to persuade the wounded soldier to return, Odysseus arranged for a young boy, Neoptolomus, to accompany him on the mission. Before arriving at Lemnos, Odysseus and his companion had discussed the difficulties that could arise because of Philoctetes' anger at being betrayed. They expected possible resistance to having his bow and arrows taken away. During the dialogue, Neoptolomus defined the meaning of virtue in relation to honesty and being true to oneself, and Odysseus justified the art of lying as a means to achieve the desired result. He spoke from the perspective of "my country right or wrong" and intended to convince the boy to resort to an untruth in regard to their deceptive goal.

Initially, Neoptolomus attempted to gain Philoctetes' trust by telling him that he also had been angry with the Greeks and disagreed with the punishment. Although this behavior reflected some of Odysseus' manipulation, it did not negate the boy's pledge to his own integrity. Distrustful at first, the injured man finally relented and they established a bond. While having a sudden seizure, Philoctetes relinquished the bow and arrows to Neoptolomus, thus leaving himself vulnerable without any defense.

When Odysseus attempted to take away the weapons knowing that Philoctetes would not leave without them, the boy refused to assist him because of his empathy for the wounded man's suffering. At that moment, a pronouncement from the gods came down from above, stipulating that if Philoctetes returned, his wound would be healed. On arrival to Troy, he recovered and the Greeks achieved victory. The story has significance in that by recognizing another's pain, and through empathy and compassion, healing can occur.

Replete with symbolism, the Greek myths reveal how unexpected trauma severely impeded such characters as Chiron and Philoctetes. Although both sustained leg wounds which deterred their mobility, they endured pain, isolation, and suffering until transforming their wounding.

WOUNDING AND HEALING

Some speculation has arisen as to whether people can truly heal others through their own wounding or trauma. A more limited point of view asserts that what accounts for the wounded healer phenomenon is "nothing other than knowledge of the wound in which the healer forever partakes" (Kerenyi, 1959, p. 99). This response however, would seem to explain only part of the issue. Early on, Buber (1965) emphasized the mutuality of healing within therapeutic relationships, which he identified as "I-thou." In this way, both parties saw the other person as a reflection of self, as opposed to "I-it" relationships in which one views the other as separate and apart. Nursing theorists Patterson and Zderad (1988) have incorporated Buber's principles into a more encompassing framework proposing the therapeutic relationship as "I-thou; I-it-all-at-once" (p. 111). Their work, described as humanistic nursing, points out that the nurse must relate to the patient as "I-thou" and observe their relationship "I-it" as it unfolds in the moment.

Another theory that helps enlighten the wounded healer concept examines the phenomenon of countertransference, originally espoused by Sigmund Freud and Carl Jung. Although the term usually appears in the treatment of psychiatric disorders, it has relevance for healing encounters in general. Since separation of the mind-body cannot truly exist, purely psychological applications of countertransference become obsolete. Most experts cite two perspectives, the classical and the totalistic, the latter being more pertinent in studying the wounded healer.

Freud briefly referred to countertransference as something unconscious, undesirable, and pathological to be "overcome" and "checked" (Gorkin, 1987; Miles, 1993). In the classical interpretation, the focus was on the practitioner's unconscious emotional reactions to a patient, reflecting unresolved conflict and describing healers who are wounded but do not recognize their woundedness (Miles, 1993). Curiously, this perspective on countertransference has been accepted by most health care professionals, although it does not adequately explain the wounded healer dynamic.

The totalistic view of countertransference would seem to be more relevant to the wounded healer in that it defines a practitioner's entire emotional response, both conscious and unconscious to the patient (Miles, 1993). Ferenczi, one of Freud's colleagues, believed that patients become intuitively aware of the analyst's actual feelings, blind spots, and neuroses, a view which allows a greater role for countertransference than what Freud advocated (Gorkin, 1987).

Discussing therapeutic work, Jung identified "insight" as an awareness of the wounding, an endurance for suffering to examine it, and the action needed to transform and transcend it (Hollis, 1989). He even suggests that those suffering from neuroses demonstrate the abnormal behavior because they have not as yet interpreted its meaning. At times, however, bearing a wound can be so painful that the healing processes may be difficult to endure when the rhythm of the patient's thoughts and actions are incompatible with the greater natural flow of the body and life in general.

According to Epstein (1994), suffering impels individuals to become more acutely conscious of themselves as well as of the isolated, denied, or repressed waves of energy. Pain, therefore, can lead to the realization that their feelings do not connect to the values that they want to guide their lives. So central have these tenets been to the work of Jung that analysts following his tradition perceive themselves to be wounded healers from the outset of their training, and they believe that suffering must be understood and transcended for growth to occur. Consequently, Jung (1913) urged health care professionals to explore their own wounds openly, emphasizing the futility of remaining secretive. In his view, patients could somehow look into the souls of healers and determine how they handled their own problems and whether they practiced what they preached (p. 198).

Greek mythology and psychoanalysis have provided us with the groundwork for more intense scrutiny of the wounded healer by other psychological theorists such as Guggenbuhl-Craig (1971), Groesbeck (1975), May (1985) and Sedgwick (1994). Questions surface as to why practitioners require knowledge of their own trauma and the need to share it repeatedly to heal, as well as how these factors relate to their awareness and participation in the healing process of patients (Groesbeck, 1975).

Groesbeck (1975) believes that healers and their patients have complementary roles, which may not necessarily be conscious. If the practitioner's task has been to facilitate a person's inner healing capability, how can it be accomplished? Contact with the wounded healer requires explanation at a deep level, with the practitioner expected to assume the patient's wounds and experience them profoundly through his or her own wounding. When achieved, the healer's response will be projected to the patient and awaken the inner healer.

Groesbeck (1975) further claims that the process energizes the patient's powers of strength and healing. Guggenbuhl-Craig (1971) has suggested that in addition to the wounded healer, a "healer-patient" archetype is stimulated each time a patient becomes ill. This observation implies that although patients seek outside healing agents, their own capacity to heal, or "inner healer," has to be activated for healing to take place (pp. 89–91).

Sedgwick (1994) emphasizes that the work of the wounded healer extends beyond empathy. Here again, we recognize that for the wounded healer to emerge, the practitioner must experience the patient's wounding, and the deeper the better. If countertransference is to emerge, the healer must reflect the capacity to be wounded so that a parallel woundedness exists. In such situations, the traditional view of empathy might be considered more superficial than in a relationship in which the wounded healer dynamic prevails and a "superempathy" emanates. Without question, the practitioner should feel the intensity of the patient's wound in the moment (Sedgwick, 1994).

When the person does not seem to heal, an interpretation must follow with some circumspection. Is the extent of healing not likely or visible at the time of the interaction? Has healing been equated with curing? Or, for example, is the death of a loved one able to bring together an estranged family with a more global healing to take place? And, can it be conjectured that the expected result may come at a future time as the person progresses toward healing? All these aspects of the healing spectrum must be pondered to stimulate transcendence of trauma and the emergence of the wounded healer.

IMPACT OF SHAMANISM ON THE WOUNDED HEALER

The process of transformation and creation of the wounded healer can be demonstrated through the ancient practice of shamanism (Dossey, 1989). Shamans predicate their therapeutic outcomes on the belief of the patient in being healed rather than on the actual techniques employed. As indigenous practitioners, they deliberately alter their consciousness through prayer, trances, and even mood-altering drugs, to obtain knowledge and power from the "spirit world," and use the insight gained to heal tribal members (Krippner, 1988).

In certain cultures, the focus of shamanic healing might have little or no bearing on the disappearance of physical symptoms but rather on becoming whole or in harmony with the community, the planet, and the person's private circumstances (Achterberg, 1988). Shamans helped patients search for the meaning of illness in their lives and to integrate it into the context of their entire being (Krieger, 1981). They became models of healing because of an openness to work at physical, emotional, and spiritual levels, as well having the ability to expand their own consciousness and transform themselves (Harner, 1988; Krieger, 1981; Achterberg, 1988; Watson, 1999). Although similar to mind healing, shamanism is perceived as more encompassing since it requires the healer to experience the patient's pain and understand how to promote the healing response more effectively.

Achterberg (1988) has asserted that becoming the wounded healer arises from some crisis that creates a personal transformation or spiritual awakening and ultimately generates the wisdom resulting in marked insight to help others (p. 117). This realization could change the perception of healers and guide them to become more knowledgeable about healing. Shamans therefore represent wounded healers in the fullest sense because they enter into and assume the patient's wounds and illnesses, transcending them by their force and power (Miller & Baldwin, 1987). They perceive woundedness as an indication of wisdom, providing insight, not as a sign of self-vulnerability (Remen, May, Young, & Berland, 1985).

Shamanic healers have often displayed their wounds as evidence of the authenticity of their healing powers derived directly from the wounding (Remen, May, Young, & Berland, 1985). Their ability to move between the worlds of the well and the ill has also been validated by the wound. As in the case of Chiron, shamans who have survived trauma are often identified as the greatest healers because overcoming the wounding itself becomes the open door to healing power and the knowledge underlying it.

Being physically disabled or afflicted with a serious disease, recovering from an addiction, or having a handicapped child are only some of the wounds that have befallen healers (Achterberg, 1988). Take the example of Don José Rios, a Huichol Indian born in the late nineteenth century who lived in the Mexican Sierras. Before losing his right hand in an accident, he had been a successful farmer and regarded his trauma as a call from the spirit world (Krippner, 1988). Also known as *Matsuwa* (pulse of energy), Don José claimed that the *Kauyumari* or Little Deer Spirit had taught him how to heal the sick. He offered prayers to the spirits, drew impurities from patients' bodies, and balanced their energy fields by using his prayer arrows. In addition to ingesting the peyote, a hallucinogenic plant to induce visions that helped him diagnose the person's illness, he prescribed treatments such as prayers, herbs, fasting, or even referral to a physician (Krippner, 1988).

A major goal of Don José's healing methods was not only to achieve his patients' recovery from illness, but also to help them find meaning and joy in their lives. As his story reveals, shamans represent the archetype of wounded healers because in most situations a crisis leads them into expanded consciousness and the will to heal. An awareness that humans are wounded by the very nature of being in the world, has stimulated a revived interest in the practices of shamans by contemporary health care practitioners who aim to broaden existing treatment approaches (Doore, 1988).

The Nurse as Shaman

Since nursing and shamanism reflect a holistic base in their approach, many nurses employ shamanic practices in furthering relationships with their patients. Their concern has been with helping people to alleviate stress and suffering from emotional, physical, and spiritual symptoms. Both groups use considerable symbolic and practical counseling to create positive attitudes and encourage self-responsibility (Krieger, 1981).

Another example of the similarity of nursing and shamanism occurs in the use of meditation and centering prior to implementing energy healing practices, such as Therapeutic Touch, Healing Touch, AMMA Therapy or Reiki. These modalities conjure up images of the shaman who often uses trancelike states of consciousness. According to Wolinsky & Gordon (1986), a trance may be described as a shrinking or fixating of attention, with its most striking feature a reduced outward attention and an inward focus, thus fixating the consciousness to a narrow frame of concentration (Erickson & Rossi, 1976). Like the shaman, nurses must be prepared before treating the patient. In the process of TT, they center themselves both physically and psychologically, conceptualizing that they represent open systems of energy and become aware of a quiet, focused, and attentive inner space (Heidt, 1981). This activity appears to simulate a trancelike state.

In some nursing circles, practitioners support the idea that the work of the shaman embodies the feminine principle exemplified by intimacy, touch, and a mutual acceptance within the healing arts (Krieger, 1981; Watson, 1999). Jung (1973) has also emphasized that the symbolic influence of the mother figure may induce humanness, compassion, and wisdom in children. These qualities tend to foster tenderness, concern for enduring values, strong religious feelings, sensitive responses to intuitive knowledge, and curiosity about the riddles of the universe (Krieger, 1981, p. 14).

WALKING WOUNDED OR WOUNDED HEALER?

Although the interpretation of the wounded healer indicates a complex phenomenon, differences should be noted when applying the term "walking wounded." The latter term, which encompasses people from all walks of life including health professionals, refers to those who have experienced trauma without understanding its affect on them. In her description of a phenomenon called woundology, Caroline Myss (1997) alludes to the walking wounded as persons who recognize that they have wounds but cannot transcend them. As she succinctly concludes, "Defining ourselves by our wounds, we burden ourselves and lose our spiritual and physical energies and open ourselves to the risk of illness" (p. 7).

Sometimes the difference between the walking wounded and wounded healer can become almost blurred when the individual makes progress on the path to transformation. In this light, consider the example of Diana, Princess of Wales. Surely, she showed this potential but died tragically before she could transcend much of her suffering. Many of the problems that appeared to confront her as she approached adulthood seemed to have stemmed from earlier years when she was abandoned by her mother. As she recalled later, "I always felt very different from everyone else, very detached. I knew I was going somewhere different, but had no idea where" (Morton, 1998, p. 34). Despite this deeply rooted woundedness she began to show signs of growth. Reflecting on the effect of her parent's divorce, she noted, "It helped me to relate to anyone who is upset in their family life. . . .I understand it. Been there, done that" (Morton, 1998, p. 36).

Abandonment represented a core personal issue for Diana, resulting in a bulimic eating disorder which was intensified by the pressures of her position when she married into the royal family. An inability to cope with her problems led to a number of suicide attempts until she realized the destructive nature of her illness: "I think the bulimia actually woke me up. I suddenly realized what I was going to lose if I let go" (Morton, 1998, p. 85). This awakening produced a positive outcome for Diana who became involved in worthy causes, such as visiting underserved areas with serious social and health problems and comforting patients with HIV infection and AIDS. Her altruistic activities suggest that she was beginning a transition, moving toward more favorable goals and resolution of her wounding.

To what extent the Princess fully recognized and integrated the dynamics of her early trauma, we will never know because of her premature death. Prior to the tragedy, however, she had already made a decision to cut back on her public life to concentrate on private matters, possibly to reflect on her life. Yet, the depth of her wounding and how it affected her behavior remains open to question, and some investigators have indicated that perhaps she suffered from a more serious pathological illness (Bedell-Smith, 1999). Whatever the motivation for her desire to help others, it can be speculated that she was in the process of developing as the wounded healer.

In professional circles, it would be erroneous to apply the term walking wounded to the wounded healer because healing does not necessarily encompass the entire human body, mind, and spirit, nor does wounding by itself create a wounded healer. Nouwen (1972) explains that making one's wounds a source of healing requires a constant willingness to recognize self-pain and suffering as rising from the depth of human suffering, which all human beings share. Becoming a wounded healer, therefore, implies that trauma must be pondered for its personal meaning and that it must be transformed and transcended.

Examples of the walking wounded may not be as rare as people in the helping professionals think. Gonsiorek (1995) suggests that sexual misconduct remains an old problem unresolved for centuries. Thus, although some cases are reported in the press, a strong possibility exists that many more such incidents are never exposed. In clergy communities, involving all denominations, some prominence has been given to accusations of molestation of younger members of their congregations (Fortune, 1995). The same behavior has also surfaced in the fields of psychotherapy and nursing when practitioners pursue an intimate relationship with patients. If untreated, the depth of the healer's wounds will not only expand within the individual, but will also exacerbate the recipient's pain.

Less extreme examples, but nevertheless poignant, can be found among health care workers who neglect to care for themselves properly. Without awareness, they drain their healing energies, making themselves therapeutically ineffective and incapable of transcending their own wounding. Practitioners who smoke or experience weight problems, such as marked obesity, have difficulty concealing their trauma from patients. The inability to provide positive role modeling of self-care hinders the performance of the healer.

Without question, the larger society as well as health professionals may also be the culprits in reinforcing the vulnerability of the wounded. Portraying himself as a wounded healer, David Smith (1999), a former clergyman, relates a compelling narrative about his own transformation. By the time Smith was fifteen, his family had relocated several times, triggering feelings of social and intellectual inadequacy and causing his school grades to fall below average. As an adult, he suffered from the death of his first child and eventually a divorce.

After becoming an Episcopal minister, Smith describes how he acquired a dominance-control attitude toward healing by purposely distancing himself from parishioners. Because of his position in the church and a sense of control within organized religion, he claimed to be superior to others. Obsessed with his power, he abandoned his wife and children emotionally and suffered a mental breakdown which required institutionalization. During that period, his wounding intensified when a church representative requested that he renounce his priesthood.

As a result of his hospital experience, Smith noted that he could detect healers who were wounded but had not transcended their trauma. He further indicated that because many of the caregivers did not seem to be particularly therapeutic, it was uncomfortable to share his problems with them. In his mind, he concluded that they projected a dominance-control-shame attitude that did not help his recovery. His tragic plight, however, eventually led to a deep self-awareness, which helped him fully comprehend and later write about the essence of the true wounded healer.

Seeking guidance, Smith turned to Carl Rogers'(1980) client-centered approach as a basis for transcending his own wounding. He learned that individuals have within themselves the means to develop self-understanding and alter their self-concepts, basic attitudes, and self-directed behavior. Such resources could be tapped in a climate fostering unconditional positive regard, congruence, and empathetic understanding, the components that represent the foundation for becoming a wounded healer (Rogers, 1980).

By practicing congruence in the health professions, surely the more nurses act naturally in relationships, the greater the probability of promoting change. Too often, an air of professionalism in the guise of cool reserve (even when inner warmth exists) may create defensiveness in the patient sensitive to the practitioner's behavior. For example, think about nurses who mechanically ask patients how they are feeling without really listening. Perhaps the practitioner has a personal or health problem or is preoccupied for some other reason. Whatever the distraction, patients can often sense when a nurse is not truly interested.

Unconditional positive regard, another quality inherent in the wounded healer may be difficult for some caregivers to practice because human nature tends to be critical at times and judgmental of others. When nurses are angry, upset, or have a family history of a certain illness, it can affect how they relate to their patients. Take the example of Martha, who works on a surgical unit where some of the patients have a history of narcotics addiction. When they approach her for pain medication, she usually delays their dosage. In her conscious mind, Martha labels the patients as "manipulative" and "drug seeking" without realizing that her attitude stems from a former serious relationship with an addicted man whom she expected to marry. Because of the hurt created by an unresolved personal problem, Martha is unable to give unconditional positive regard to her patients and remains wounded.

According to Rogers (1980), empathetic understanding relates to the caregiver's skill in accurately recognizing patients' feelings and personal meanings and in knowing how to communicate them. Sedgwick (1994) builds on this interpretation with the idea of "superempathy," in which not only must understanding take place but also the ability to go beyond the spoken word and analyze the meaning in relation to the patient's experience.

With empathy underlying the nurse's therapeutic use of self, a subsequent transformation into the wounded healer can evolve predicated on the level of consciousness attained within helping relationships. Unless change occurs, the healer will remain wounded in the symbolic cave in a state of suffering like Chiron before his descent into Hades. Although the trauma an individual endures may be ever present and in various stages of healing, the painful residual can be diminished.

SELF-AWARENESS: THE KEY TO HEALING

Newman (1986) points out that opening and expanding an individual's awareness leads to the possibility of self-healing. This view may explain the difference between remaining wounded and becoming the wounded healer, which is attained through increasing levels of consciousness. True healing emerges when a fresh view of the person's life and problems reaches a clearer focus, releasing the body's energy, and repatterning disharmony to reflect a higher degree of wellness.

We might ask how realistic is it to study such an intangible concept as consciousness? Wilbur (1993) discusses this idea within a spectrum containing a number of overlapping bands or levels, such as the ego, the existential, and the level of the mind. As the first level, the "ego" refers to the perceptions individuals have of themselves including the conscious, unconscious, and intellect. Since many healers, such as nurses and physicians function at this level, their performance is limited by their unrealistic approach in attempting to live up to an idealized professional image. A common manifestation includes the "perfect nurse," clad in an impeccably neat, white starched uniform, who effortlessly treats each patient with a smile and superficial pleasantness. Because such individuals cannot possibly achieve the unrealistic goals set for themselves, they will be ineffective healers with a limited impact on their surroundings.

Not until nurses become more seasoned and enter into the professional world are they more likely to recognize their own wounding. All too often, as with students in preparatory programs, there is no secure place or opportunity for them to explore feelings that arise in clinical situations. If not encouraged, however, consciousness regarding personal and professional wounding remains at the ego, or most superficial level of awareness, as illustrated in the following scenario.

During a psychiatric rotation in a general hospital, Anna, a 20-year-old nursing student discovered that when she arrived on a locked unit, the patient whom she had previously cared for had become seriously disturbed that day and was transferred. As a result, the clinical instructor, Linda Hall, assigned her to Frances, another patient, who appeared to be quiet and unassuming at first. After Anna spoke to Frances, the woman suddenly started to yell, cursing and ranting about rape and murder. Frightened, the student rushed out of the room to the nurses' station, sat down, and sobbed.

When the instructor located her, Anna could not explain her feelings and declared that she was a "bad nurse" for not being able to handle the situation with Frances. Believing the difficulty was related to impaired communication, Ms. Hall realized the need for some problem solving as well as closure for both student and patient. She then shared some of Frances' history including rape at an early age; she also related that Frances' violent language reflected feelings that the patient had been unable to process.

After the explanation, the instructor asked Anna if she would return to Frances, but the student remained fearful and unaware of what was causing her reaction. When Linda Hall offered to accompany her, Anna agreed, and when they entered the patient's room, she calmly apologized for her behavior. Frances then seemed to be comforted and felt less abandoned by the student's actions. As a consequence, Anna showed some growth even though at the time she lacked an in-depth awareness of the personal dynamics contributing to the incident.

During the nurse-patient interaction, Anna's consciousness remained at the ego level in relation to the existing situation. Upon probing by Ms. Hall after leaving Frances, Anna realized that the encounter had reminded her of verbal abuse from both her parents and teachers in childhood.

Unlike the more superficial ego level, the "existential" level of consciousness refers to the total organism, including the soma and the psyche, as well as how persons perceive themselves. It also enables the individual to recognize separateness and distancing from outside experiences. Thus, practitioners who operate at this level do not limit themselves merely to the "professional" images indoctrinated in them as students, but rather incorporate the totality of their lives in their work. By demonstrating these attributes within the helping relationship, they draw on feelings along with intellect as a basis for practice which facilitates the healing process.

Ruth's story exemplifies the existential level of consciousness. As the daughter of holocaust survivors and an experienced psychiatric nurse, she is a somewhat anxious individual and reluctant to take risks. At the same time, she possesses a high level of self-awareness, personal identity, and a positive professional image. A single woman in her mid-forties, Ruth can be sociable, but tends to spend most of her time either at home close to her parents or at the hospital where she has worked for the past twenty years.

One day while walking outside the institution, Ruth met Mrs. Martin, a schizophrenic patient hospitalized on her unit several times and discharged to outpatient care. At the time, the woman revealed that her seven-year-old son was exhibiting bizarre behavior, such as drawing pictures of people being mutilated and hanging themselves. When the nurse suggested that Mrs. Martin consult with her son's counselor in school, the patient resisted the idea and abruptly walked away, leaving the nurse deeply troubled by the reaction.

On later reflection, Ruth realized that outside of the hospital walls, she had neither control nor staff available to support her in guiding Mrs. Martin. At this level of consciousness, she recognized a sense of helplessness as well as aloneness in both herself and the patient. Unable to put closure to the situation, she eventually began to scrutinize what occurred within a larger context. After examining her feelings more deeply, she began to realize that her own concerns took precedent over the need to elicit more details from Mrs. Martin. The suggestion of a counselor may have been sound but premature without having sufficient information. The impromptu meeting with the woman and Ruth's eventual insight although belated, generated a positive outcome for the nurse. In time, she became more aware of her own responses to the patients in her care.

Commenting on the third level, that of the "mind," Wilbur (1993) notes that it includes the body, mind, and the rest of the universe, which Jung (1989) refers to as the collective unconscious. Dossey (1989) and others characterize it as the nonlocal mind, encompassing more than the individual's consciousness. When individuals approach this level, they may experience it as being one with the universe. Practices such as meditation and centering help healers engage in deeper thought, promoting transcendence to higher levels of consciousness.

Although the state of transcendence offers individuals new possibilities, this view has neither been widely shared nor practiced in Western cultures, which focus mainly on developing a healthy ego (Wilbur, 1993). Yet, acquiring more in-depth awareness must be considered when achieving the role of the wounded healer because it connects to a power for strengthening and healing the self and mirroring such possibilities for others.

The level of the mind may be likened to the universal energy that encompasses all human beings. Many of us tap into the mind level although unsure of the results. For example, in pygmy societies when the entire tribe believes that a person will die soon, death usually follows (May, 1989). What could account for such an occurrence, which some may view as bizarre? One explanation might be that collective forces and attitudes may exert a tremendous pressure on the dying person and that he or she simply obliges (May, 1989). Similarly, studies reveal that prayer for a seriously ill patient tends to effect recovery more fully and quickly than in cases where it has not been offered (Dossey, 1989).

Robert, a 35-year-old nurse working on a critical care unit, reported a unique healing experience reflecting expanded consciousness. While attending a 70-year-old man who had undergone a triple bypass operation, he felt compelled to give extra attention to the patient. As the hours passed, he became strongly connected to the man without understanding why. At the end of the shift, Robert received news that his father had undergone emergency heart surgery in a hospital over 3,000 miles away, precisely at the time that he was taking care of the critically ill man. He perceived this event as a manifestation of a greater consciousness resulting from being more open to his own feelings in his practice.

Robert's interpretation of the situation can be viewed as credible because he experienced consciousness at the level of the mind that might have involved clairvoyance or mental telepathy; others, however, may attribute it to mere coincidence. Certainly, receptivity to such possibilities within nurse-patient interactions should be considered in helping nurses to provide more appropriate care.

An individual's level of consciousness has relevance to one's ability to become a wounded healer which depends on several factors such as (1) degree of awareness regarding the effects of trauma on healing relationships or the level of the ego, (2) ongoing consciousness of feelings, thoughts, and actions and their effect on others at the existential level, and (3) the integration of how woundedness can be used in healing at the level of the mind including psychic healing.

Although wounding occurs in various degrees and affects people differently, the imperfection of being human creates a wound in itself. As stressed earlier, the very nature of the trauma does not determine whether or not an individual becomes a wounded healer, but rather the person's recognition of the traumatic event along with the willingness to accept and transcend it.

NURSING AND THE WOUNDED HEALER ARCHETYPE

The wounded healer archetype can help nurses to transmit recuperative power to patients who ultimately heal themselves regardless of the modality used. Using themselves therapeutically, they recognize their own patterns and remain open to the possibilities of further growth. For example, nurses in recovery from compulsive overeating realize that such recovery is a lifelong process and can draw upon this insight to impart greater understanding to an obese patient.

Focusing on the patient's needs represents an essential component of the healing process. Therefore, in order to awaken the wounded healers in themselves, nurses must examine their attitudes toward each healing encounter itself. Does the approach ascribe to a reductionistic or holistic view, or to a combination of both? Is the type of healing sought by the patient essentially material, spiritual, psychological, social, or multifaceted? How flexible is the relationship with the patient and what are the mutual expectations? And if nurses have been recovering from an illness similar to the patient's, is their focus on caring for the person or on gaining emotional support for themselves, or perhaps both?

Of marked importance is the ability of nurses to use past trauma to heal others rather than to use the clinical situation as a vehicle for resolving their own problems. During nurse-patient interactions, this area can blur, because practitioners cannot be certain when new awareness will surface. If it happens, the thrust must be kept on the patient, and at a later time the nurse may wish to discuss his or her perceptions with an objective colleague or a professional therapist.

The healing intent, as another consideration, refers to what the nurse consciously desires to accomplish during the encounter. Factors include the healer's motivations and feelings in approaching patients as well as questions about his or her attitude. Also necessary is determining the patient's health status and willingness to change.

Finally, presence, or "being there," involves consciousness and intent; it concerns a relational style that includes "being with" as well as "doing with" (Patterson & Zderad, 1988). As with consciousness, the levels encompass the physical, psychological, and therapeutic realms, with the latter representing the most significant component (McKivergin, 2000). Although physical presence refers to body contact and psychological presence to interactions concerning the mind, therapeutic presence describes the nurse as relating to the patient as a whole being, using all the resources of body, mind, and spirit (McKivergin, 2000).

By its very nature, nursing incorporates many characteristics of the wounded healer archetype into its own core values of caring, compassion, and empathy. Nurses serve as instruments of healing when they create an openness within themselves to enhance the opportunity for another to feel secure, bring disharmony into alignment, and gain the capacity to heal by sharing their authenticity and unconditional presence to help remove any barriers to the healing process. (Montgomery-Dossey, Keegan, & Guzzetta, 2000). Although nursing has generally been perceived as a "doing therapy," such as administering medications and other forms of material healing, it remains primarily a "being therapy" (Montgomery-Dossey & Guzzetta, 2000, p. 11). The nurse's therapeutic use of self remains the major expression of the wounded healer through consciousness, intention, and being present.

SUMMARY

The roots of wounding in Greek mythology illustrate the meaning of suffering and its relationship to the wounded healer. Among prominent theoreticians such as Jung, the recognition exists that trauma should be exposed as well as explored for its interpretation by the practitioner and patient. Although he and Freud believed in the phenomenon of countertransference, they espoused different approaches to apply within therapeutic relationships. Other theorists from the more modern school of thought have offered telling insights into the use of congruence, self-awareness, and empathy in the healing encounter.

A notable observation is the similarity between nursing and shamanistic practices stemming from ancient times. Holism is an important philosophical and pragmatic component of the techniques employed by both traditions in their aim to balance body, mind, and spirit. As a complex concept, the wounded healer has been erroneously equated with the walking wounded, who undergo trauma without understanding its impact. Conversely, people who transcend their own wounding have developed the capacity for consciously incorporating it into the healing process, which is the true mark of the wounded healer.

DISCUSSION GUIDE

1. Give three examples of countertransference in nursing practice.
2. Discuss how nursing practice resembles shamanism.
3. What are the major differences between "walking wounded" and "wounded healer?"
4. Describe the significance and relationship of the three levels of consciousness to healing.
5. What are the core elements in Carl Rogers' client-centered approach? How do they relate to becoming a wounded healer?

REFERENCES

Achterberg, J. (1988). The wounded healer: Transformational journeys in modern medicine. In G. Doore (Ed.), *Shaman's path: Healing growth and empowerment* (pp. 115–129). Boston: Shambala.

Bedell-Smith, S. (1999). *Diana in search of herself: Portrait of a troubled princess.* New York: Random House.

Buber, M. (1965). *Between man and man* (R. G. Smith, Trans.). New York: Macmillan. (Original work published 1937)

Doore, G. (Ed.). (1988). *Shaman's path: Healing growth and empowerment.* Boston: Shambala.

Dossey, L. (1989). *Recovering the soul: A scientific and spiritual search.* New York: Bantam Books.

Early, E. (1993). *The raven's return: The influence of psychological trauma on individuals and culture.* Wilmette, IL: Chiron.

Epstein, D. (1994). *The 12 stages of healing: A network approach to wholeness.* San Rafael, CA: Amber-Allen.

Erickson, M., & Rossi, E. (1976/1980). Two level communication and microdynamics of trance. In E. Rossi (Ed.), *The collected papers of Milton H. Erickson on hypnosis and suggestion* (pp. 430–451). New York: Irvington.

Fortune, M. (1995). Is nothing sacred? When sex invades the pastoral relationship. In J. C. Gonsiorek (Ed.), *Breach of trust: Sexual exploitation by health care professionals and clergy* (pp. 29–40).Thousand Oaks, CA: Sage.

Gonsiorek, J. C. (Ed.). (1995). *Breach of trust: Sexual exploitation by health care professionals and clergy.* Thousand Oaks, CA: Sage.

Gorkin, M. (1987). *The uses of countertransference.* Northvale, NJ: Jason Aranson.

Groesbeck, C. J. (1975). The archetypal image of the wounded healer. *The Journal of Analytical Psychology, 20,* 120–145.

Guggenbuhl-Craig, A. (1971). *Power in the helping professions.* New York: Spring.

Harner, M. (1988). What is a shaman? In G. Doore (Ed.), *Shaman's path: Healing, growth and empowerment* (pp. 7–15). Boston: Shambala.

Heidt, P. (1981). Scientific research and Therapeutic Touch. In P. Heidt and M. A. Borelli (Eds.), *Therapeutic Touch* (pp. 3–12). New York: Springer.

Hollis, J. (1989). The wounded vision. *Quadrant, 22* (2), 25–36.

Hover-Kramer, D. (2000). Relationships. In B. Montgomery-Dossey, L. Keegan, & C. E. Guzzetta (Eds.), *Holistic nursing: A handbook for practice* (pp. 639–658). Gaithersberg, MD: Aspen.

Jung, C. G. (1913). The theory of psychoanalysis. In H. Read, M. Fordham, G. Adler, and W. McGuire (Eds.), *The collected works of C. G. Jung.* (CW4) Bolligen Series XX. Princeton: Princeton University Press.

Jung, C. G. (1973). Four archetypes. (R. F. C. Hull, Trans.) *Bollingen Series XX* (pp. 7–14). Princeton: Princeton University Press.

Jung, C. G. (1989). *Memories, dreams and reflections.* New York: Vintage. (Original work published 1963)

Kerenyi, K. (1959). *Asklepios, archetypal image of the physician's existence.* New York: Pantheon.

Krieger, D. (1981). *Foundations for holistic health nursing practices: The renaissance nurse.* Philadelphia: Lippincott.

Krippner, S. (1988). Shamans: The first healers. In G. Doore (Ed.), *Shaman's path: Healing growth and empowerment* (pp. 101–114). Boston: Shambala.

May, R. (1985). The wounded healer. In *Perspectives in nursing, 1985–1987* (pp. 3–11). New York: NLN.

May, R. (1989). The empathetic relationship: A foundation of healing. In R. Carlson and B. Shield (Eds.), *Healers on healing* (pp. 108–110). New York: Penguin Putnam.

McKivergin, M. (2000) The nurse as an instrument of healing. In B. Montgomery-Dossey, L. Keegan, and C. E. Guzzetta (Eds.), *Holistic nursing: A handbook for practice* (pp. 207–227). Gaithersberg, MD: Aspen.

Meier, C. A. (1967). *Ancient incubation and modern psychotherapy.* Evanston: Northwestern University Press.

Miles, M. W. (1993). The evolution of countertransference and its applicability to nursing. *Perspectives in Psychiatric Care,* 29 (4), 13–20.

Miller, G. D., & Baldwin, D. C. (1987). Implications of the wounded healer paradigm for the use of self in therapy. In M. Baldwin (Ed.), *The use of self in therapy* (pp. 139–151). Binghamton, NY: Haworth.

Montgomery-Dossey, B., Keegan, L., & Guzzetta, C. E. (2000). *Holistic nursing: A handbook for practice* (3rd ed.). Gaithersberg, MD: Aspen.

Morton, A. (1998). *Diana: Her true story.* New York: Pocket Books.

Myss, C. (1997). *Why people don't heal and how they can.* New York: Harmony.

Newman, M. (1986). *Health as expanding consciousness.* St. Louis: Mosby.

Nouwen, H. (1972). *The wounded healer.* New York: Image.

Patterson, J. G., & Zderad, L. T. (1988). *Humanistic nursing.* New York: NLN.

Remen, N., May, R., Young, D., & Berland, W. (1985). The wounded healer. *Saybrook Review,* 5 (1), 84–93.

Rogers, C. (1980). *A way of being.* Boston: Houghton Mifflin.

Rose, H. J. (1960). *A handbook of Greek mythology: Including its extension to Rome.* New York: Dutton.

Sedgwick, D. (1994). *The wounded healer: Countertransference from a Jungian perspective.* London: Routeledge.

Smith, D. (1999). *Being a wounded healer: How to heal ourselves while we are healing others.* Madison, WI: Psycho-Spiritual Publications.

van der Post, L. (1975). *Jung and the story of our time.* New York: Random House.

Watson, J. (1999). *Postmodern nursing and beyond.* New York : Churchill Livingstone.

Whan, M. (1987). Chiron's wound: Some reflections on the wounded healer. In N. Schwartz-Salant & M. Stein (Eds.), *Archetypal processes in psychotherapy* (pp. 197–209). Willmette, IL: Chiron.

Wilbur, K. (1993). *The spectrum of consciousness.* Wheaton, IL: Quest.

Wolinsky, S., & Gordon, M. (1986). *Trances people live: Healing approaches in quantum psychology.* Fall Village, CT: Bramble.

CHAPTER 4

TRAUMA: ROOTS AND REPERCUSSIONS

Never shall I forget that nocturnal silence which deprived me, for all eternity, of the desire to live. Never shall I forget those moments which murdered my God and my soul and turned my dreams to dust. Never shall I forget these things, even if I am condemned to live as long as God Himself. Never.

Elie Wiesel, Night

What are the dynamics underlying the healing process and the wounded healer in relation to the effects of a traumatic event or wounding? Are these occurrences identical or do certain differences become apparent? Whereas the term "wound" describes a type of injury, "wounding" generally indicates how it occurred. Although wounding and trauma result from an unfortunate happening, the latter tends to connote a more intense and serious outcome. At a more superficial level, both can be reduced to physical, psychological, emotional, social, or spiritual components. Whatever the source, the injury can profoundly affect the individual and have long-term repercussions.

As health care providers, nurses must be willing to examine the issues surrounding trauma and wounding. If we deny or reject the possibility that these can occur in ourselves as well as others, it will seriously hamper our ability to heal. Although exposure to painful, traumatic situations may be difficult to face, repression or avoidance of the problem becomes a formidable obstacle to the potential for healing. Without question, health professionals are often exposed to disturbing situations in their practice that can leave them with psychological scars. Unfortunately, among the top five causes of nurses' deaths, suicide may be at least six times higher than in the general population (Belanger, 2000). The risk for addiction may also be higher in those with unresolved trauma, and can precipitate suicidal behavior.

Trauma assumes more prominent visibility when it involves the sudden death of a loved one, such as in the case of the TWA airplane crash over Long Island in 1996 or the earlier ill-fated flight of the Challenger space shuttle. More common examples appear in individuals who incur serious injuries from automobile accidents or fires, causing them permanent disability and disfigurement. More often than not, however, are the hidden or undetected consequences of traumatic events resulting from domestic violence, child abuse, or even the effect of neonatal trauma related to premature birth. Regardless of the underlying cause, traumatized individuals often suffer silently and require the support of able caregivers to achieve satisfactory resolution of their problems.

THE NATURE OF TRAUMA

A useful way to understand more clearly the nature of trauma may be to relate it to the image of a black hole, in which the sufferer feels trapped and despondent (van der Kolk & McFarlane, 1996). In such a circumstance, a black hole in space represents a bottomless pit with gravity pulling all matter into its domain, including light. When individuals cannot identify the root of their pain, their response is similar to being drawn into a black hole with little hope or possibility of escape.

Herman's (1992) interpretation bears some relevance to this phenomenon when she notes that trauma "overwhelms the ordinary system of care that gives people a sense of control, connection, and meaning" (p. 33). By suppressing traumatic feelings, depression and the unconscious reenactment of certain patterns can begin to surface, whereas the ability to release such emotions has a greater potential for aiding recovery. When coping with trauma, whether a single event or an ongoing pattern, several factors need to be considered, including the age at which the injury occurs, the subsequent energy drain, and the person's inner strength in dealing with it.

When a sudden resurgence of traumatic memories happens, it may create confusion and even fear because recollections do not necessarily reflect coherent, linear thought processes, and may be related to how the individual coped with the original trauma. If the memories have not been integrated and accepted, they can plague the victim through bodily sensation rather than thoughts or feelings. For example, a young boy who has been scratched by a thorny plant may experience some numbness in his arm at a later time when seeing a similar plant, even though he does not necessarily associate it with the original causative agent.

We may question to what extent, if at all, a person can realize consciously the source of wounding as well as how to deal with it effectively. Levine and Frederick (1997) point out that an energetic "trauma residue" may become trapped in the body-mind after the wounding occurs. Contrary to the belief that a stimulus or triggering event can precipitate the reliving of trauma, they claim that it is actually the inability of the system to discharge the energy that causes the residual to remain frozen. Their view seems similar to the way Chinese medicine and other Eastern traditions perceive illness as energy stagnation within the body-mind, and if unexpressed, the trauma generates physical or emotional pain, or a combination of both.

To understand traumatization, nature provides us with some useful clues (Levine & Frederick, 1997). Of interest is that when animals in the wild become threatened, they freeze or are immobilized before being attacked by a predator, and as an adaptive response, it may save their lives. After attacking an antelope, a cheetah frequently drops its prey while dragging it to another place to devour it. Thus, there still may be a chance for escape by assuming a submissive stance.

In animal life, the act of freezing has the tendency to alter the mind-body state physiologically so that pain is not experienced. If the animal escapes, it quickly passes through this state and returns to its normal everyday activities. When human beings undergo trauma, the response becomes locked within the body and remains there unless discharged; otherwise, anxiety and depression will result.

Ironically, it may not be the nature of the wound itself but rather the reaction to it that increases the intensity. Brennan (1993) refers to the notion of "image conclusion" or the way individuals view themselves to explain post-traumatic patterns. If a person has been abandoned repeatedly early in life, he or she may draw the conclusion, "If I love, I will be abandoned," a belief that will color similar future experiences (p. 6). Unless this perception is connected to its real meaning and brought into awareness, a type of desertion trauma pattern remains and manifests in various life events. Not uncommonly, people attract dating partners or spouses who eventually forsake them.

According to Davidson & Jackson (1985), long-standing hidden symptoms of trauma that occur in some nurses and other health care professionals may be intergenerationally transmitted. In the case of a nurse reared by a parent obsessed with dying, the individual may undergo a heightened sense of death anxiety when caring for critically ill patients. Another example can be found in Holocaust survivors who relate their concentration camp experiences in great detail and later their children develop psychological disturbances of varying kinds.

Esther, a nurse with the latter background, became interested in trauma nursing and alleviating the pain of others. As a child, she learned of her mother's ordeal of having been in a concentration camp and liberated at the age of thirteen. Subsequently, Esther's family moved often, always living in basement apartments because her mother feared that the captors would return. Her desire to become a trauma nurse represented an attempt to undo the intergenerational pain she had unknowingly inherited.

Bowen's (1985) family systems theory affirms that emotional and behavioral patterns can be transmitted from one generation to the next. Trauma may also have a cumulative effect on the individual especially if the pattern seems to "skip a generation." To illustrate, as in cases of alcoholic grandparents, the behavioral symptoms relating to addiction can be passed down to the children who keep it a family secret and do not drink themselves. Although they appear normal in most respects, other addictive attitudes and responses such as perfectionism or workaholism may appear.

These behavioral patterns as described, may confuse the grandchildren who sense that something is wrong; yet the source of the problem (intergenerational addiction) has never been brought out in the open (Smith, 1988). If they, in turn, resort to substance abuse, the family's denial unfortunately robs them of awareness that could prevent continuation of the destructive cycle. Bradshaw's (1995) succinct observation sums up the dilemma when he states, "It's what you don't know that can hurt you" (p. ix).

As noted in the earlier black hole image, the effects of trauma can place an individual in emotional isolation, comparable to a cocoon. Figure 4–1 below shows the wounded child archetype, often associated with the emotional life. In this depiction, the adult face seems agonized on the surface of what appears to be the superficial layer of the skin. Underneath, the child looks expressionless or numb, tightly wrapped in what seems to be a follicle or capsule, and appears comfortable and protected while the adult above bears an anguished expression. From this description, it can be compared to a skin irritation that erupts, which becomes more painful than after it begins to drain.

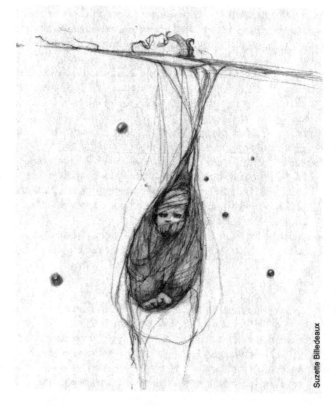

Figure 4–1 The Child Goes into Hiding
The Child Goes into Hiding (Whitfield, 1991, p. 28). (Reprinted with permission).

Trauma often stays buried because of the fear of pain in opening the wound even though relief can be anticipated. Additionally, the body-mind tries automatically to protect the person who feels discomfort and may not understand the nature of the threat. Therefore, an overwhelming, unresolved childhood occurrence can surface with the same degree of emotion that existed at the time of the original wounding. For example, when an abused child reaches adulthood, unrecognized traumatic feelings can reappear if triggered by reminders. Unfortunately, the inability to express such feelings early in life and the energy generated by these feelings give wounded individuals the sense that they will be devastated by revealing the trauma.

Evolution of Wounding into Trauma

Since people respond to a traumatic episode in different ways, to what can we attribute the variations in the ways in which wounds are interpreted, expressed, and processed? What factors operate for a simple wound to evolve into trauma? Suppose a homemaker accidentally cuts her hand while opening a can of salmon that causes a small irritation on the skin. If the injury does not heal quickly and becomes infected, it can lead to deleterious consequences. What began as *simple* wounding therefore can become a traumatic event such as a systemic infection and even hospitalization. Although the incident may consciously fade in time, whenever the woman opens other cans of food, she may become anxious, even fearful. Unless she has an awareness of the origin of the wounding and its subsequent traumatic results, the same painful responses will continue to emerge.

As shown in the above example, the original wound was more or less benign in nature at the outset. For reasons differing in individuals, the process of wounding can range from simple to complex. Perhaps the homemaker's immune system was compromised at the time of the injury, or there may have been a more covert reason for the infection to occur. Although it may seem farfetched, another possibility could be that with a divorce in progress, she expressed her emotional pain through the physical wound because of an inability to verbalize her feelings.

Another example of wounding evolving into trauma may be illustrated through the long-time practice of performing tonsillectomies with ether as the choice of anesthetic. Administered by a cone over the face, it left some youngsters with a fear of suffocation. Fortunately, the procedure was of short duration and in time the pronounced smell of the drug and the feeling of being unable to breathe tended to fade. Yet, other symptoms could have eventually developed such as dreading crowds or enclosure in confined spaces like elevators. Years later, however, these individuals may recall having gone through the earlier ordeal but without connecting their present phobia to any prior trauma.

It is evident that a traumatic event may differ from the way it manifests itself, or for that matter, how or when it is remembered. Although most wounds such as a simple scratch are considered inconsequential, they can interfere with an individual's equilibrium. When left unattended, they send a distress signal to which the body-mind may respond with a more serious illness.

The intensity of the wounding also determines the level of trauma and the potential for healing. In cases of abuse, contributing factors include the degree and duration of parental dysfunction and mistreatment; gender of the dysfunctional parent; severity of parental codependence; personality of the child and his or her perception of the family dysfunction; the presence and severity of chemical dependence; and stress and cultural factors (Whitfield, 1991). Psychological or emotional wounding that progresses to traumatic wounding leaves the person with feelings of inadequacy and can perpetuate additional dysfunctional behaviors aimed at healing. Since the problem remains hidden, the trauma stays intact and adds another layer, such as addiction, to an already overstressed system.

STRESS AND ITS IMPACT

Trauma may be perceived as a stress derived from a more serious type of blow to the integrity of the body-mind than a minor wound, and as such, lodges in the system and drains what Myss (1997) refers to as a "cellular bank account" (p. 16). The term corresponds to Selyé's (1974) general adaptation syndrome (GAS), in which only a certain amount of energy exists within the system, either used or conserved throughout life. Observing that not all stress should be viewed as negative, Selyé (1974) classifies two types. He characterizes "eustress" as the general stimulation needed to survive, which produces increased energy and a sense of well-being, and "distress," which depletes the individual's coping strength.

Stress can be considered essential in that it contributes to health or illness; without it, the organism will not survive. The repeated responses appearing at frequent intervals over a period of time convert into lifestyles, demonstrated by certain behavior patterns (Achterberg & Lawlis, 1980). Pert (1997), a neurobiologist who addresses the importance of the body-mind, discovered the opiate receptor in the early 1970s. Her research pioneered the study of how neuropeptides and their receptors act to orchestrate many key bodily processes, linking behavior and biology to ensure smooth functioning of the organism.

In general, receptors are typically proteins anchored in the outer cell membrane with a site that can bind with substances such as drugs, hormones, or neurotransmitters. This process modulates the chemical processes of the cell and communicates information to other cells which in turn become altered. Pert (1997) concludes that many areas of the brain associated with emotion, as well as specific cells in the immune system, become enriched with various neuropeptide receptors.

Her observations suggest that neuropeptides and their receptors join the glands and immune system in a network of communication between the brain and the body, representing the biochemical substrate of emotion. Claiming

:hat these receptors exist for a reason, (prior to the advent of mood-altering drugs interacting with them), she further notes the importance of the individ-ual's biochemistry and how it can create or modify the emotional state.

Nursing and Stress

Nursing has been one of the first professions to set standards for "rape trauma syndrome," a cluster of symptoms that frequently occurs after sexual assault. Yet, even with their proclivity for recognizing trauma in others, nurses often have difficulty in seeing themselves as victims. At the organiza-tional level, their struggle to professionalize over the years has created marked wounding leading to an inability to deal with the stressors that con-tinually plague the field.

Sometimes, professionals cannot be easily convinced that they have been wounded, and working in stressful health care environments only reinforces the trauma. During the 1980s and 1990s when hospitals and other agencies stream-lined their operations through reorganization, restructuring, and employee ter-minations, such actions created a state of mental and emotional withdrawal in many of the workers affected (Noer, 1993). Not only did staff trust in the insti-tutions dissipate, but nursing care also suffered from a lack of proper resources.

Stress places a heavy toll on caregivers even under the best of circum-stances. A wound that persists can fester and lead to serious repercussions such as burnout and traumatic stress. Burnout has been characterized as be-ing caused by a constant focus on others, a perceived lack of control over one's circumstances, and the inability to participate in major work decisions (Sum-mers, 1992a). Traumatic stress emerges when dominant negative feelings and behaviors are reawakened and reinforced in the health care setting, generat-ing more severe symptoms. On the other hand, when individuals can accept their feelings, they acquire a positive approach and thereby can avoid dis-tressful consequences.

In studying nurses with psychotrauma, Buyssen (1996) proposes that the degree of traumatization relates to vulnerability and protective risk factors. Being vulnerable to becoming traumatized depends on the degree and dura-tion of exposure to the precipitating event, individual or family history of psy-chiatric problems, anticipation of the occurrence and degree to which it can be controlled, strong identification with the victim, and imagined guilt related to the happening. Conversely, protection from severe traumatization involves the expectation and controllability of the circumstance, personal adaptive coping style, and social support.

Progression of Trauma to Posttraumatic Stress Disorder (PTSD)

Recognized initially after World War I, combat fatigue and shell shock were terms freely used to describe a set of symptoms associated with the severe stress of battle. Not until the Vietnam War, however, was the diagnosis of posttraumatic stress disorder (PTSD) introduced in lieu of earlier terminology. Complex and more prevalent than realized and resulting from severe wounding, PTSD has been defined as various psychological and biological responses to an acute stressor experienced directly or indirectly as well as chronically (Symes, 1995). Symptoms may appear shortly after the event, lasting less than a month, or may surface gradually, remaining for an indefinite period. Convinced that Florence Nightingale suffered from PTSD as an aftermath of her experiences in the Crimean War, some authorities have portrayed her as "a bereaved, haunted woman who paced endlessly up and down in her room at night, sleepless and withdrawn" (Harbart & Hunsinger, 1991, p. 385).

According to van der Kolk & McFarlane (1996), PTSD essentially represents a "failure of time to heal all wounds" (p. 7). Shalev (1996) corroborates the conclusion of Levine and Frederick (1997) that the disorder demonstrates an inability to recover from mental traumatization or to take the steps necessary to release traumatic memory from the mind-body complex. For resolution to take place, human beings require an awareness as well as a knowledge of the dynamics underlying the trauma.

This observation may be particularly applicable to uninformed or misinformed health professionals about the frequency of trauma and its connection to the physical and emotional symptoms of patients along with their own reactions in the clinical setting. Unfortunately, caregivers are often led to assume in their training that they can handle existing traumatic situations, without knowing the repercussions of a potential stress disorder (Harbart & Hunsinger, 1991).

An awareness of PTSD requires recognition as well as understanding of its more prominent manifestations, such as persistent intrusions of memory, compulsive exposure to situations reminiscent of the trauma, attempts to avoid triggers of trauma related emotions, and an inability to effectively modulate their arousal. Accompanying the condition may be problems with sustaining attention, distractibility, and alterations in psychological defense mechanisms and personal identity (van der Kolk & McFarlane, 1996). According to Tomb (1994), PTSD is frequently triggered by everyday happenings rather than primarily by the stress of combat.

Intrusive Thoughts and Feelings

The intrusion of traumatic memories, ranging from flashbacks and intense emotions to somatic sensations or nightmares, produces symptoms particularly disturbing to the individual who cannot discern the underlying cause. What then can account for such a reaction? More than likely the timeless and fragmented nature of the memories are embedded in the sufferer's trauma as a contemporary experience instead of belonging to the past (van der Kolk & McFarlane, 1996). This feature of PTSD may have special significance for nurses in that we consistently face traumatic experiences in our daily practice when personal reactions arise while caring for affected patients.

For example, alcoholics and drug abusers represent a wounded population, having endured the consequences of their addiction along with society's disapprobation. When health care providers are exposed to such individuals, some respond with anger and indignation, which can be interpreted as a release of their traumatic residue. Because they lack the necessary insight, their own unexplored wounding remains in the unconscious and will then be reinforced.

Blair & Ramones (1996) point out that it is not unusual for professionals dealing with traumatized patients to experience "violent, disturbing dreams, to become paranoid, hypervigilant and overconcerned with their own safety, or to experience severely disruptive symptoms such as intrusive thoughts, sleep disturbances, phobias, aversions and dissociate reactions" (pp. 24–25). Emphasizing the contagious nature of wounding, Crothers (1995) asserts that hospital staff may begin to show PTSD symptoms with a resurfacing of their own dormant traumatic memories.

Traumatic events can be recent such as an earthquake, which the individual has read about but has not encountered, or such occurrences can stir up hidden past wounding. To illustrate, take the case of Gloria, a nurse assigned to care for a battered baby in the emergency room. Her exposure to the infant triggered repressed feelings of a childhood experience in which she was physically abused by her mother. Gloria suddenly froze at the thought of attending the baby and after experiencing severe queasiness, asked a staff member on the unit to assume her responsibility for the child.

In this situation, the nurse's behavior demonstrated emotional withdrawal that prevented her from performing therapeutically in the care of the child. Her reaction however, reflected a pattern that began years earlier when subjected to parental mistreatment. Although Gloria didn't understand her behavior, she felt guilty about approaching another colleague. That night she began to have nightmares about being assaulted. In time, she decided to avoid any contact with children and requested a transfer to an adult medical unit. Since the nature of the wounding remained buried and thus unresolved, a strong possibility existed of her having flashbacks and intrusive thoughts related to the original trauma.

Trauma Reenactment

A major yet paradoxical aspect of PTSD occurs with trauma reenactment in which wounded people unconsciously place themselves in a situation reminiscent of a past traumatic episode. Nowhere can this be better exemplified than with abused women who either remain with their perpetrators or leave them only to find new partners with similar destructive behavior patterns. Many of the victims relate a history of battering in their families of origin and unconsciously seek the same experiences in adult relationships. Because of erroneous conditioning, abuse frequently becomes equated with love (Celani, 1994). In such situations, all too often the blame regrettably falls on the individual being abused.

Addressing how trauma reenactment affects nurses, Summers (1992b) refers to *the chase*, in which caregivers pursue relentless traumatic memories in the corridors of hospital and medical offices. She explains that they become part of a "plot" revolving around their own pain, unaware of the driving force behind it. Individuals continually reach the climactic scene where the opportunity to heal presents itself, but cannot use it for this purpose until they understand consciously the dynamics of the chase.

As an example, Millie, a nurse working on a clinical unit, tended to form relationships with alcoholic patients and to date them socially after discharge. Unaware that her behavior stemmed indirectly from the emotional abuse inflicted by her alcoholic father in childhood and her sense of helplessness at the time, she attempted to control the alcoholic patient to counteract an unresolved sense of powerlessness.

A type of reenactment trauma frequently observed in nurses is that of parentification, where their oversolicitous care can become counterproductive to themselves. This pattern represents a form of role reversal in which parents inappropriately depend on children to care for their emotional or physical needs (West & Keller, 1991). It often occurs in families with a history of substance abuse, depression, and other dysfunctional behaviors. Parentified children employ "overcaregiving" as a primary means of relating to others.

In adulthood, parentification may progress to compulsive caretaking of others at the expense of one's self. Bowlby (1977) points out that such adults are unable to receive care: They must always be the ones to give it and ignore caring for themselves. Their frustration can lead to a sense of shame, guilt, and inferiority.

It is not surprising that nurses traumatized by parentification express it as a means of exerting control when caring for others in clinical settings. Even though caregiving and accountability represent desirable traits for nursing practice, they must be balanced to produce a healthy outcome. In situations where nurses assume the responsibility for a patient's behavior instead of allowing the individual to take the initiative, the problem continues to be unresolved and recidivism follows. Without an awareness of the dynamics involved in the relationship, they may become angry and frustrated when the patient returns repeatedly.

Avoiding Triggers of Trauma-Related Emotions

Certain attempts to avoid triggers of trauma-related emotions can generate emotional or psychic numbing, a key aspect of PTSD. Patients who follow this pattern often become detached from others including their families. In addition, they may lose interest in their surroundings, report an inability to feel normal emotions, and often believe that death is imminent (van der Kolk & McFarlane, 1996). This type of avoidance has been aptly described as being "behind a glass wall" (Herman & Schatzow, 1987, p. 6).

Nora, a community health nurse, became interested in sports medicine with a determination to keep herself physically fit. Both of her brothers had muscular dystrophy, which created marked emotional and financial hardship on her parents. Being the only physically healthy sibling, she became exceedingly distressed being around her brothers since it caused sadness and severe guilt feelings. Unable to cope with the circumstances, Nora ultimately decided to visit her family infrequently and concentrate on her own health.

When reaching extreme proportions, efforts to avoid trauma-related emotions can lead to isolation. In such cases, the individual may become housebound or emotionally removed in an effort to shut out memories or dreams of the trauma and sometimes the people associated with it (Tomb, 1994).

Although we like to think of nursing as a "people to people" business, some nurses cannot communicate comfortably with their patients. For example, Elizabeth, a staff nurse on an oncology unit, appeared quite detached from the people in her care. Yet, like some nurses who begin to avoid patients that they are initially drawn to care for, she failed to comprehend that she was reenacting her own trauma. Although unaware of it, her behavior stemmed from a denial of a past experience when a younger sibling died in early childhood from leukemia. Not until the cause of Elizabeth's difficulty had been brought to the surface and she transcended her wounding was she able to relate effectively to oncology patients.

Hyperarousal and Attention Problems

It is not surprising that wounded individuals become more highly aroused or hypervigilant. When trauma has a long duration or is cumulative, the aftereffect may become harder to control. Common behavior difficulties arise, including sleep disturbances, anger outbursts and exaggerated startle responses, problems in concentrating, and progressive deterioration in social, occupational, or other areas of functioning (Shearer & Davidhizar, 1995).

Excessive stimulation of the central nervous system at the time of the injury may result in alterations in brain chemistry producing mood changes and other negative symptoms (van der Kolk, 1996, p. 214). States of hypervigilance and hyperarousal can be easily detected in the behavior of some health care professionals, especially when years of caring for traumatized patients have weakened their coping mechanisms. Their stress becomes intensified when combined with sleep deprivation and the constant physical and emotional demands of patients who may be fearful, angry, and troublesome (Harbart & Hunsinger, 1991).

Alterations in Psychological Defense Mechanisms and Personal Identity

Does trauma have an impact on an individual's defense mechanisms and persona, and if so, how is it manifested? In cases of abuse and violence, the victim will usually undergo a change in self-perception that often requires cognitive and emotional therapy (van der Kolk & McFarlane, 1996). Nurses are all too familiar with the reactions of colleagues who will not admit their fear of being out of control when exposed to or physically threatened by violent patients. What can account for this response, which to some might be viewed as courageous and as "unnatural" to others?

Perhaps behavior of this nature has its basis in a childhood of abuse when to show fright or resistance could mean further physical harm. As a consequence, the person assumes a demeanor of extreme calm or indifference even when unwarranted. More perplexing is that this type of distortion in personal identity can lead to a trauma reenactment when wounded individuals unconsciously place themselves or others in potentially hazardous surroundings, reminiscent of the distant injury. The following scenario demonstrates such a situation.

Late one afternoon, Maureen, the nursing care coordinator, and Vinnie, a male social worker and the program director of an inpatient substance abuse unit, were talking in his office when suddenly they heard a loud noise coming from the day room. They hurried to investigate and saw Lena, one of the counselors, crying and holding the side of her face covered with blood. She had been attacked by Eddie, a former patient visiting the unit who was intoxicated and being restrained by two inpatients.

While waiting for hospital security to arrive, Maureen expressed marked dismay that an act of violence could happen on her unit. Anger and feelings of helplessness overwhelmed her as she saw Eddie sobbing and in seconds lashed out at him repeatedly shouting, "I want you out of here, I want you out of here!"

As soon as she spoke, Maureen regretted her sudden outburst, feeling ashamed for losing control and showing such rage at a former patient. At the time, she did not realize that her reaction stemmed from a pattern beginning as a teenager when her father drank heavily and often became violent. During these episodes, she would demand that he leave the house.

Maureen's response to Eddie stunned Vinnie and the other staff members since she had always remained composed in crisis situations. They responded by withdrawing from her, emotionally unable to provide any support. As a result, she felt abandoned by the team, which added to her wounding. McFarlane & van der Kolk (1996) point out that wounded persons suffer a second injury if not supported by the people they count on. When censured for creating their own traumatic situations, victims experience shame and disgust by their failure to prevent what has occurred. Another unfortunate consequence is that exposure to a traumatic happening of victims becomes hazardous to the mental health of those closest to them (Crothers, 1995).

THE RECALL OF TRAUMA

How critical is it to unearth a wounding long buried within the unconscious mind? Are some people better off when certain traumas are not disturbed or raised to the surface? Addressing these profound and delicate questions depend on many factors.

It should be noted that throughout human development, all body responses are recorded at both conscious and unconscious levels making memories *potentially yet not always* accessible to coherent recall. Whitfield (1995) asserts that traumatic memories remain stored in long-term memory and may not always be easily identified and remembered. Furthermore, when they emerge, the person may not understand or recognize them. It is not uncommon for fragmented or incomplete elements of the event to appear and thus cloud the true meaning with denial and attempts to forget the past that become the hallmarks of psychotrauma (Whitfield, 1995).

The degree of trauma or developmental stage at which it has occurred undoubtedly affects the interpretation attributed to the memory and how it has been processed. For example, although traumatic memories at the preverbal stage may be recalled, attempting to discern as an adult what they meant seems improbable since no words existed at the time of the original experience. Survivors with the most severe memory deficits have been amnesic of the particulars when the abuse occurred, yet often report the most "jarring recurrent, intrusive symptoms such as flashbacks and body sensations" (Courtois, 1988, p. 298).

Because the meaning of a happening may change over time with inner life events coloring the experience, accurate recall may not be possible. A lack of cognitive, coherent memory, however, does not negate the past occurrence. Although no specific event may generate a traumatic response, the root of the problem may stem from a pattern of abuse when the victim was violated as a child on many levels. Unraveling the pattern in adulthood, however, can become a long and arduous process.

Does relating a traumatic event to another individual help resolve the problem? A compelling question indeed, requiring some consideration. At what point has the event been communicated? Immediately following it, or months or even years later? And in whom does the affected person confide? A family member, friend, or professional person?

Whether people share a traumatic experience depends on their capability to remember and communicate it. In addition, can their perceptions be validated by the observations or empathetic understanding of another? A physically mistreated child will be able to resolve the wounding more quickly when he or she can confide in a trustworthy adult, who will accurately determine the veracity of the situation and implement actions of a protective nature to prevent the trauma from progressing to PTSD.

As Whitfield (1995) notes, an abusive environment does not always lend itself to encouraging children to feel secure enough to talk about painful experiences or feelings. Therefore, the likelihood of disclosure diminishes and the potential is reduced for healing the wounding at an earlier stage. In cases where individuals have undergone an isolated traumatic incident such as rape later on in life, the victim may be more apt to share the event if no prior pattern of abuse existed.

Another important consideration concerns the utility of recall. Rather than remember, abused children may find it easier to forget trauma through dissociation, repression, or suppression (Whitfield, 1995). Bodily sensations or feelings may also surface as memory of the event. Ellenson (1985) has observed perceptual disturbances and somatic hallucinations occurring in all adult female incest survivors. Such trauma that goes untreated is often manifested by suffocating or gagging sensations.

Without question, trauma recall may be induced by exposure to similar, associated, or anticipated events. Consider the phenomenon of vicarious traumatization or transforming the inner experience of a health care provider that occurs from empathizing with a wounded client (Pearlman & Saakvitne, 1995). Whether or not nurses have undergone identifiable trauma in their lives, they may become affected by graphic stories that clients relate. Repeated contact with the darker side of human nature or what Jung (1989) refers to as the *Shadow* can influence dramatically the psychological processes of others, since it becomes the reflection of the self. He characterizes the *Shadow* as the inferior being within ourselves, wanting to perform all those things that we consciously view as undesirable or repulsive.

It can be speculated that some nurses and other caregivers may have been attracted to the helping professions by the very nature of their personal wounding. Whatever the reason for their choice, many positive features can emerge when they develop a conscious realization of their own wounding and then become valuable participants in providing care. The calling to help others may not even be recognized as a need to revisit and reenact traumatic situations.

Unfortunately, sporadic reports appear about the behavior of health professionals, including nurses, who commit heinous acts against their patients. In fact, there have been cases where the effects of trauma are revealed in the person's violent behavior. Hickey (1997) proposes that childhood trauma serves as a triggering mechanism for serial murderers when they cannot cope with life events, the most common being rejection from parents and relatives (p. 87). Far too often, these perpetrators have little insight into the origin of their wounding, which may come from the lack of human feeling exhibited repeatedly by their abusers. In turn, serial killers experience no emotional connection with their victims and continue their criminal patterns without remorse.

Two such cases involved Terri Rachals, a registered nurse, and Michael Swango, a physician, who were accused of committing murder. Although viewed by many as productive individuals, personal and intergenerational trauma seems to have accounted in part for the destructive roles they played in society. In 1986, Rachals who worked in a Georgia hospital, was indicted on six counts of murder and twenty counts of aggravated assault due to alleged poisonings of patients through lethal injection of potassium chloride (Hickey, 1997). Previously, she had been viewed as an excellent intensive care nurse, active in church affairs, and described by neighbors as the "last person one would suspect of harming anyone" (p. 220).

Confessing to the crimes, Rachals was diagnosed as competent to stand trial after psychiatric evaluation. Her traumatic past revealed that she had been molested by her stepfather and suffered from "blackout periods" unable to remember what she said or did during those episodes. Found by a jury to be mentally ill and guilty in only one case of aggravated assault, she was sentenced to 17 years in a Georgia prison.

Michael Swango's story paints a chilling picture of a Midwesterner and son of a Vietnam veteran who abused his family and preferred spending nine years at war to being home. From an early age, young Michael appeared to have been traumatized by parental physical and emotional mistreatment and through intergenerational trauma by a fascination with violence. His mother reinforced his dysfunctional behavior by helping him put together a scrapbook containing stories of hideous events.

Eventually Michael went to medical school where many of his colleagues noticed that he exhibited a cool indifference to patients and their families. After becoming a physician, he was convicted of poisoning his fellow ambulance drivers and spent time in prison. After his release, however, he obtained employment as an emergency room physician even though evidence of his criminal history was available. When reports appeared about a number of suspicious, untimely patient deaths (even witnessed), it took years before the authorities caught up with him (Stewart, 1999). Finally admitting his guilt, Swango was convicted in September 2000 and sentenced to three successive terms of life imprisonment without possibility of parole. Throughout his court appearance, he showed no shame or regret.

In situations reflecting severe trauma, such as in kidnappings or torture, sometimes the victim may identify with the aggressor in a phenomenon characterized as the Stockholm syndrome (Hickey, 1997). First described in 1973, it came into prominence when four Swedish people, held as hostages in a bank vault for six days during a robbery, became attached to their captors. Another example that received wide coverage in the American press involved the heiress Patty Hearst, kidnapped in 1974 by the Symbionese Liberation Army (SLA). Some months later, she renamed herself "Tanya," joined the ranks of the SLA, and assisted them in a bank robbery. Years later and rehabilitated, Hearst was pardoned for her complicity when she was able to convince others that she joined the group after torture and brainwashing (Martin, 2000).

According to some psychologists, the Stockholm syndrome occurs when the victim bonds to the perpetrator as a survival mechanism. An analogy can be made to situations in everyday life when battered women become attached to their partners even though they are threatened with abuse and possible death if they attempt to leave. In the health care community, nurses fearful of jeopardizing their financial security continue to work in inconsiderate or abusive institutions.

Rx for Healing

On the surface, the healing of psychic wounds may appear to be a simple process but it requires considerable energy that is neither visible nor experienced consciously. Wounding of this nature has often been more difficult to identify and treat than that associated with physical trauma. Although a traumatic agent may be recognized, the actual body-mind response becomes integrated, and therefore not only the cause but the individual's reaction to it will affect the degree of trauma and the ability to heal.

Claridge (1992) proposes some techniques for retrieving and integrating traumatic memory as well as beginning the process of healing. She emphasizes educating individuals to understand that recall will take place in response to similar situations occurring in the present. By listing events that trigger strong feelings, the patient and practitioner might be able to ascertain the nature of hidden wounding. In some cases, a story or newspaper article can stimulate a reaction that generates clues about the traumatic event. Claridge (1992) recounts an incident involving a female patient who became upset on seeing a news broadcast about a child trapped in a well. The program ignited a recollection of being imprisoned in her home as a form of childhood abuse.

Myss (1997) contends that healing cannot occur until completing the unfinished business of the past. She cites the existence of unresolved or deeply consuming emotional, psychological, or spiritual stress as the primary pattern underlying physical illness. Included among the factors that determine the presence of illness are not being able to give or receive love; a lack of humor and an inability to distinguish serious concerns from the lesser issues in life; and a lack of control over their own lives especially when it means compromise or altering plans or flexibility.

Other considerations involve the degree to which individuals care for their physical well-being and the absence or loss of meaning in life. Myss (1997) observes that some people become ill as a form of denial to escape their problems. She explains that when persons can identify and address certain patterns arising from their own wounding, innate health may be awakened and healing fostered.

Wounding of the Nursing Profession

Is nursing a wounded profession, and if so, what are some of the dynamics behind this observation? Numerous facets add to the complexity of the issue, which has historical roots that cannot be overlooked. Certain stereotypes still pervade in American society, such as the image of the paternalistic physician and the compliant nurse.

Beyond the health care arena, turf problems between men and women have existed for decades although the women's movement launched in the late 1960s has been an impressive step forward. Yet, nurses, the largest group of female health professionals, continue to lack the visibility and power necessary for making a significant impact nationwide.

Although nursing has attempted to professionalize over the years, as evidenced by trends in higher education and research involvement, its lesser prepared rank and file, which constitutes the majority of practitioners, continue to play a subservient role. A positive force has been the growing interest in alternative approaches to care by nurses involved in holistic practice, which generates more practitioner and patient satisfaction than functioning under the medical model with its focus on curing alone.

The social and cultural patterns that affect women and other susceptible groups tend to build trauma into everyday life, producing outcomes that inhibit the expansion of energy for self-development. Nurses may be particularly vulnerable to this outcome by virtue of their sex since the majority are female. Furthermore, as an oppressed group within the health care hierarchy, they may experience abuse not only from the medical establishment and hospital administration but also, in some situations, from one another, which can rekindle latent personal trauma.

Muff (1988) discusses the roots of nurses' wounding in relation to both personal and professional realms and suggests that the two areas cross over. She cites identity and boundary difficulties and poor self-esteem as being partly responsible for nursing's difficulties. These factors can enhance the potential for creating trauma. Along with personal issues harbored by nurses, a parallel process occurs at the same time while practicing their profession. Just observe all the patient care functions they perform, including those outside the realm of nursing practice. As a result, a professional identity crisis can occur.

Another aspect of the professional and personal interplay is the independence-dependence bind. According to Muff (1988), this conflict is fueled by the need of nurses to be there for others and a reliance on others for self-esteem, which makes the separation process more difficult. With good intentions, there sometimes exists a selflessness in nursing that involves undervaluing one's self and overvaluing others in the name of caring (Muff, 1988). Such a pattern however, represents the essence of the personal wounding that has failed to advance from the walking wounded stage to that of the wounded healer.

SUMMARY

The roots of trauma may or may not be visible, making it a more frequent occurrence than generally believed. Because nurses and other health care providers suffer from unrecognized wounding in their personal and professional lives, they need to develop some awareness for the purpose of their own health as well as that of their patients. Otherwise, if unresolved, trauma generates undesirable outcomes that can create posttraumatic stress disorder. The process involves understanding the intrusions of traumatic memories, trauma reenactment, avoiding triggers of trauma-related emotions, and other PTSD manifestations.

From Nightingale's time to the present, nurses have been subjected to various traumatic events that entail internal conflicts as well as those from outside forces. By virtue of its history and the fact that nursing remains essentially a profession of women, the potential for traumatization and its intergenerational transmission strongly exists. Personal and professional healing will prevail through self-recognition and the ultimate transcendence that characterizes the wounded healer.

DISCUSSION GUIDE

1. Describe the factors in which stress can precipitate the emergence of trauma.
2. Identify the ways that wounding can progress to posttraumatic stress disorder.
3. Wounding of the nursing profession has several manifestations. What is the historical significance and its aftermath?
4. Explain why nurses are prone to vicarious traumatization.
5. Identify how nurses can begin to recognize trauma in their own lives.

REFERENCES

Achterberg, J., & Lawlis, G. F. (1980). *Bridges of the bodymind: Behavioral approaches to health care*. Champaign, IL: Institute for Personality and Ability Testing.

Belanger, D. (2000). Nurses and suicide: The risk is real. RN, 63 (10), 61–64.

Blair, D. T., & Ramones, V. (1996). Understanding vicarious traumatization. *Journal of Psychosocial Nursing*, 34 (11), 24–34.

Bowen, M. (1985). *Family therapy in clinical practice*. New York: Jason Aronson.

Bowlby, J. (1977). The making and breaking of affectional bonds. *British Journal of Psychiatry*, 130, 201–210.

Bradshaw, J. (1995). *Family secrets: What you don't know can hurt you*. New York: Bantam.

Brennan, B. A. (1993). *Light emerging: The journey of personal healing*. New York: Bantam.

Buyssen, H. (1996). *Traumatic experiences of nurses: When your profession becomes a nightmare*. London: Jessica Kingsley.

Celani, D. P. (1994). *The illusion of love: Why the battered woman returns to her abuser*. New York: Columbia University Press.

Claridge, K. (1992). Reconstructing memories of abuse: A theory based approach. *Psychotherapy*, 29 (2), 243–252.

Courtois, C. (1988). *Healing the incest wound*. New York: Norton.

Crothers, D. (1995). Vicarious traumatization in the work with survivors of childhood trauma. *Journal of Psychosocial Nursing*, 33 (4), 9–13.

Davidson, P., & Jackson, C. (1985). The nurse as survivor: Delayed post-traumatic stress reaction and cumulative trauma in nursing. *International Journal of Nursing Studies, 22* (1), 1–13.

Ellenson, G. S. (1985). Detecting a history of incest: A predictive syndrome. *Social Casework, 66,* 525–532.

Harbart, K., & Hunsinger, M. (1991). The impact of traumatic stress reactions on caregivers. *The Journal of the American Academy of Physicians Assistants, 4* (5), 384–394.

Herman, J. L. (1992). *Trauma and recovery: The aftermath of violence from domestic abuse to political terror.* New York: Basic Books.

Herman, J. L., & Schatzow, E. (1987). Recovery and verification of childhood sexual trauma. *Psychoanalytic Psychology, 4* (1), 1–14.

Hickey, E. W. (1997). *Serial murderers and their victims* (2nd ed). Belmont, CA: Wadsworth.

Jung, C. G. (1989). *Memories, dreams and reflections.* New York: Vintage. (Original work published 1963)

Levine, P., & Frederick, A. (1997). *Walking the tiger: Healing trauma.* Berkeley, CA: North Atlantic.

Martin, J. (2000). *A look back at Patty Hearst.* ABCNEWS.com

McFarlane, A. C., & van der Kolk, B. (1996). Trauma and its challenge to society. In B. van der Kolk, A. C. McFarlane, & L. Weisaeth (Eds.), *Traumatic stress: The effects of overwhelming experience on mind, body and society* (pp. 24–46). New York: Guilford.

Muff, J. (Ed.). (1988). *Women's issues in nursing: Socialization, sexism and stereotyping.* Prospect Heights, IL: Waveland. (Original work published 1982)

Myss, C. (1997). *Why people don't heal and how they can.* New York: Harmony.

Noer, D. M. (1993). *Healing the wounds: Overcoming the trauma of layoffs and revitalizing downsized organizations.* San Francisco: Jossey Bass.

Pearlman, L., & Saakvitne, K. (1995). *Trauma and the therapist: Countertransference and vicarious traumatization in psychotherapy with incest survivors.* New York: Norton.

Pert, C. B. (1997). *Molecules of emotion: The science behind body-mind medicine.* New York: Touchstone.

Selyé, H. (1974). *Stress without distress.* New York: Signet.

Shalev, A. Y. (1996). Stress versus traumatic stress: From acute homeostatic reactions to chronic psychopathology. In B. van der Kolk, A. C. McFarlane, & L. Weisaeth (Eds.), *Traumatic stress: The effects of overwhelming experience on mind, body and society* (pp. 77–101). New York: Guilford.

Shearer, R., & Davidhizar, R. (1995). Hidden scars: Post Traumatic Stress Disorder. *Nursing Connections, 8* (1), 55–63.

Smith, A. W. (1988). *Grandchildren of alcoholics: Another generation of co-dependency.* Deerfield Beach, FL: Health Communications.

Stewart, J. B. (1999). *Blind eye: The terrifying story of a doctor who got away with murder.* New York: Simon & Schuster.

Summers, C. (1992a). Nursing stress: Burnout or PTSD. *Revolution, 1,* 40–46.

Summers, C. (1992b). *Caregiver, caretaker: From dysfunctional to authentic service on nursing.* Mt. Shasta, CA: Commune-a-Key.

Symes, L. (1995). Post traumatic stress: An evolving concept. *Archives of Psychiatric Nursing, IX* (4), 195–202.

Tomb, D. A. (1994). The phenomenology of post-traumatic stress disorder. *Psychiatric Clinics of North America, 17* (2), 237–250.

van der Kolk, B. (1996). The body keeps score: Approaches to the psychobiology of posttraumatic stress disorder. In B. van der Kolk, A. C. McFarlane, & L. Weisaeth (Eds.), *Traumatic stress: The effects of overwhelming experience on mind, body and society* (pp. 214–241). New York: Guilford.

van der Kolk, B., & McFarlane, A. C. (1996). The black hole of trauma. In B. van der Kolk, A. C. McFarlane, & L. Weisaeth (Eds.), *Traumatic stress: The effects of overwhelming experience on mind, body and society* (pp. 3–23). New York: Guilford.

West, M. L., & Keller, A. E. (1991). Parentification of the child: A case study of Bowlby's compulsive care-giving attachment pattern. *American Journal of Psychotherapy, 45* (3), 425–431.

Whitfield, C. (1991). *Co-dependence: Healing the human condition.* Deerfield Beach, FL: Health Communications.

Whitfield, C. (1995). *Memory and abuse: Remembering and healing the effects of trauma.* Deerfield Beach, FL: Health Communications.

Wiesel, E. (1960). *Night.* New York: Bantam.

CHAPTER 5

REFLECTIVE PRACTICE: FOUNDATION FOR HEALING

How nice it would be if we could only get through into the Looking-Glass House! I'm sure it's got such beautiful things in it!

Lewis Carroll, *Alice's Adventures in Wonderland*

How can health professionals acquire greater insight into themselves, expand consciousness, and become more skillful practitioners? Since it is a complex process, self-examination and its relationship to clinical practice is often not readily undertaken because it tends to revive old and often-dormant pain. Since the perfectionism of nurses usually appears to be the rule rather than the exception, the individual may find it difficult to admit errors or a less than faultless performance. If the nurse remains unaware of shortcomings, however, feelings of inadequacy and poor performance may begin to surface and impair the desired outcome.

Almost two decades ago, Donald Schön (1983), a social scientist, claimed that a crisis of confidence in personal knowledge exists when professionals fail to live up to the values and norms they espouse and that this crisis may lead to their becoming ineffective practitioners. Although adaptability is the key to creating new ways of caring for patients along with using appropriate resources, it may be problematic in a reductionistic system that focuses mainly on data and outcomes. In an effort to legitimate itself within the scientific community, nursing has moved toward objective tools such as nursing diagnosis, care plans, and care maps. In some cases, however, nurses avoid these methods because of time pressures, heavy workloads, and disinterest in approaches that seem inadequate for documenting care.

Frequently, personal and professional wounding remains unrecognized as well as unaddressed, and when exposed, it confronts resistance. Early (1993) examined the mythological reference to the raven which can be associated with the wounded healer. Symbolically, birds represent transformation and transcendence by virtue of their ability to fly. In its original state as a white bird in Native American folklore, the raven stole light from the spirit people, brought it to human beings, and then turned black as it flew through the smoke hole of the light-keeper's dwelling.

71

Greek myths also characterize the raven in a similar light, pointing out that when the bird brought unfortunate news to Apollo regarding the infidelity of Asclepios' mother, its color was immediately transformed from white into black. Early (1993) interprets this conversion as one in which the raven is punished and becomes a trauma survivor, as symbolized by the changing of its color. To extrapolate from the raven's story and express it in human terms, the transformation in people who have been wounded occurs when their trauma has been brought to the conscious level and generates new perceptions.

THE BASIS OF REFLECTIVE PRACTICE

Schön's (1983) work has laid the foundation for the study of reflective practice in recent decades. He identifies two levels, the first being *reflection-in-action* in which practitioners employ intuition to refine their interventions as they are implemented. The second level, *reflection-on-action*, requires a more conscious and systematic approach that utilizes retrospection.

Reflection-in-action focuses on behavior revealed in actions as they occur, and is similar to the process of intuitive understanding as described by Benner (1984). In her study, Benner discusses expert nurses who may possess vast amounts of information that are applicable in a clinical situation. Yet, she cites the difficulty they may have in articulating the rationale for carrying out a specific activity. At the same time, when these nurses have an intuitive grasp of the situation, they can detect and treat a problem quickly and without a great deal of deliberation (Benner, 1984). This kind of pattern develops because professionals have encountered certain clinical situations numerous times previously, and the particular cognitive steps involved in a process have been transformed into specific behavior patterns.

For example, a patient indicates difficulty in swallowing her food and has resorted to drinking protein shakes. Although medical tests reveal no disease process, the expert clinical nurse caring for this patient does not accept the explanation that the woman's problem has been due merely to anxiety. Instead, based on her past experience, she instantly "knows" that an eating disorder could be involved.

In situations using *reflection-on-action* or a "reflective conversation with the situation," health professionals develop the capability of analyzing knowledge in which they have attained significant mastery (Schön, 1983). Although new to some, reflection evolves out of the introspective process advocated early on by Wundt (1897) and Titchener (1912), who concluded that inner and outer experiences did not indicate different objects but rather differing points of view.

Titchener (1912) viewed introspective theory as encompassing two approaches. Through the use of direct introspection, the individual perceives the event in the moment and describes it immediately, whereas indirect introspection refers to recall at a later time, followed by elaboration. The introspective process aims to illuminate the state of consciousness. William James (1950), the well-known American philosopher and psychologist, interprets the nature of consciousness as a stream flowing effortlessly rather than one in a static state.

Using introspective concepts as a basis, reflective conversation involves the intrapsychic level, or self-talk, and the level of shared dialogue with other individuals. Inner dialogue is a highly subjective activity that may be incongruent with what others perceive, arising initially from a series of interactions between children and parents. If perceived in a negative light, this activity results from conversations entrenched in the mind that may be indiscernible from the present and contain certain irrational beliefs. The important consideration is not what happens to us, but how our interpretation of an activity affects our thinking and feelings (Ellis & Harper, 1975; Wolinsky, 1993).

As observers of life, human beings create their own internal worlds. Much of a person's self-concept often reflects an echoing of the voices of parents held within. Wolinski (1993) proposes that trauma patterns become embedded into the body-mind where they have been accepted and then replayed when activated. The "wounded inner child identity" emerges as traumatic material, and is assimilated into the affected youngster's psyche (p. 15).

EXPANDING CONSCIOUSNESS THROUGH SACRIFICE

Believing that many human beings lack insight into their true natures, Ouspensky (1981) suggests that to achieve higher levels of consciousness, people must discard the wounded inner child identity. Such an aim may be accomplished by sacrificing four principal patterns that inhibit self-awareness: *excessive talking, expressing negative emotions, excessive fantasy,* and *suffering.*

We have all been exposed to people who tend to chatter so incessantly that their jabbering may be characterized as compulsive behavior. Often, the pattern is manifested by repetition as well as the need to become the center of attention. Various reasons may account for the motivation behind such behavior, which tends to alienate others and intensify an individual's negative self-talk such as "nobody likes me anyway." Inappropriate self-disclosure may also occur when practitioners are unprepared to meet the needs of their patients and consequently talk about themselves to decrease their own anxiety.

The second pattern to be sacrificed, expressing negative emotions, appears in people who act as if nothing ever seems right with the world, a response that serves to ward off unpleasant feelings or situations. Although it may not be easy to identify negative reactions when expressed nonverbally, the behavior can still be present in the guise of body language such as grimacing or frowning. At the other end of the pendulum, a Pollyannish attitude may not be desirable, but continual negativity that includes criticism of others or self-abasement, incites anger and resentment. The expression of negative emotions is singularly absent in individuals secure within themselves and with their own *Weltanschauung*. Secure people display a sense of personal responsibility for their behavior and a receptivity to change.

According to Ouspensky (1981), excessive fantasy, the third pattern, negates any attempt to acquire higher levels of awareness because it takes the individual into a dream world away from reality. Fantasizers do not envision such ideals as becoming great poets, actors, or writers, but rather dream about being rescued from untenable situations like abusive marriages, unpleasant working conditions, or serious illnesses. Resorting to excessive fantasy can be dangerous, resulting in distraction and possible harm to the person or others. The best antidote involves positive visualization that includes defining future goals and the steps necessary to achieve them.

As the final pattern on the path to self-awareness, clinging to suffering may be one of the most difficult to overcome, especially for women who have assumed excessive responsibility. Holding on to the need for suffering implies overextending oneself and controlling every situation regardless of where the true accountability lies. It also appears in behavior reflecting responsibility for the happiness of others (Bepko & Krestan, 1985). Some individuals tend to adopt the persona of the long-suffering martyr, a reaction that may be applicable to nurses. For example, many practitioners find it difficult to refuse a request to work extra hours and experience guilt if unable to meet all the needs of persons in their care.

A close association exists between the pattern of suffering and the "great healer" archetype, in which professionals believe that it is their skillfulness which restores others to health. Although their caregiving may have components of goodness and generosity, when taken to the extreme it becomes an unhealthy "heal everything, fix everything compulsion that leads to dysfunctional patterns" (Pinkola-Estes, 1992, p. 283). The example that follows illustrates this problem.

As a dutiful child, "Jane" was compelled to satisfy her parents who repeatedly insisted that she be perfect, particularly in her schoolwork. This early indoctrination of the need for perfection dominated Jane in many endeavors as she approached her adult years. At both the conscious and unconscious levels, she often berated herself when unable to attain a 100 percent performance in whatever activities she pursued. Anger and guilt usually accompanied her feelings of inadequacy.

When Jane entered nursing school, one of her instructors pointed out the seriousness of making a medication error and the dire consequences for the nurse as well as the patient. Unfortunately, the student erred on one occasion and gave a patient the wrong vitamin dosage. The incident became more humiliating when the unit supervisor castigated her in the presence of the other staff. She began to reprimand herself, while the shame intensified and the episode consumed her mind.

Sometime later when Jane was about to prepare a blood transfusion at a patient's bedside, the man alerted her that the treatment was not for him. Realizing the potential error, she panicked and an uncontrollable fear overcame her. Subsequently, she began to dread work and froze at the thought of giving medications. It wasn't until she finally sought therapy that Jane could reflect on her childhood behavior and understand how she had related to her parents when she failed to meet their extremely high and unrealistic expectations. She found it difficult when she grew older to view herself as an ordinary human being with limitations and failings. Through her therapy, however, Jane developed a stronger self-awareness and her long-time pattern of suffering underwent a gradual positive change.

REFLECTION: A TOOL FOR SELF-KNOWING

Although a complex process, reflection represents a valuable tool in helping nurses to understand themselves and the work they perform. Reflection can be defined from various points of view, but the method allows thought content to be analyzed in a more systematic way without totally removing the subjective component from self-analysis. In reflecting, the person cultivates an observing "I" so as to become as objective as possible when attempting to comprehend inner experiences. Taylor (1998) emphasizes that reflection is the "key to making sense of human existence because lived experiences accumulate together and gather interpretive significance as they are remembered" (p. 141).

Willis (1999) identifies three modes of reflection as contextual, dispositional, and experiential. In the first aspect, the occurrence is looked upon in connection with location in time, space, and social context. This impression allows people to uncover the meaning of events regarding similarities and differences in everyday life. Any occurrence may be either so mundane that it goes unnoticed or so unusual that it captures the person's attention.

Jane's case described earlier can be analyzed in relation to the three modes of reflection. As a nursing student, she had not made any previous dosing errors. Therefore, her situation regarding the wrong medication as well as the transfusion could be easily identified within the context in which it occurred. In the next or dispositional mode, predisposing factors which influenced her problem could be determined. Jane had not been aware that childhood trauma emanating from the need for perfection affected her performance or that she was becoming more anxious in response to it. As a result she could not reflect on the matter at the time.

Finally, the experiential mode of reflection tends to highlight the event as it occurred in the moment. For Jane, however, reflection was not possible because of her traumatic history. With the help of a therapist, she eventually learned to process her feelings by understanding the nature of her wounding and its effects on her nursing practice.

Johns (1995) characterizes reflection as a personal experience that enables the practitioner to access, make sense of, and learn through everyday clinical occurrences that arise from conflicting values. He emphasizes that in the process, contradictions surface between what is intended to be achieved and the actual practice itself. Exposing these contradictions, he points out, can initially increase the individual's sense of frustration when seeking new ways to approach clinical situations after uncovering reflective insights (Johns, 1998). If a personal crisis occurs, it may be the moment of contradiction that becomes clear upon reflection, and eases the person's transformation into the wounded healer (Bailey, 1998).

How can individuals practice reflectively within the mistake-punishment mentality that often governs working situations, thus preventing them from becoming introspective and growing as professionals? Alluding to the biblical fable of Lot's wife, Rutter (1995), a Jungian scholar, describes the dilemma of the trauma victim who dares to face painful circumstances. In this example, the woman was turned into salt because she dared to look back and witness the destruction of Sodom and Gomorrah and the suffering of their inhabitants as they met a devastating end. Similarly, the trauma victim who has been molested may fear the emotional and perhaps even physical consequences at the hands of the perpetrator if he or she acknowledges and reports the event.

In most cases, reflecting on the trauma is the first step toward exposing the pain. Woodman (1990), another Jungian analyst, notes that the Greek myth of Perseus has been useful in depicting how addictions and other painful problems can be addressed in this way. As part of his mythic quest, Perseus, son of Jupiter and Danae, had been charged to slay Medusa, one of the Gorgons, a group of hideous female beasts with huge teeth, brazen claws, and snakes for hair. Similarly, as in the story of Lot's wife, gazing directly at these creatures would result in his being transformed to stone.

Aided by spiritual powers, Pluto's helmet of invisibility, and Mercury's winged sandals, the unseen Perseus managed to advance within striking distance. Using the reflection on Minerva's magic shield to guide his fatal blow, he attacked the monster. The story of Perseus has some significance in that although we may not be able to confront our problems directly because of their hurtful nature, we may address them in our lives by scrutinizing any repetitive dysfunctional patterns. A common example could be in cases of compulsive overeating, in which excessive food consumption may reflect unresolved emotional needs; if examined openly, the problem can diminish.

INTEGRATION OF TRAUMA THROUGH REFLECTIVE PRACTICE

Reflective practice is gaining a great deal of support in today's nursing community (Johns & Freshwater, 1998). In addition to applying it to improve practice, it can be used as an effective tool for beginning trauma integration to foster self-examination.

Among the numerous theories defining reflective practice, Paterson and Zderad (1988) cite the phenomenological approach in which human beings and their experiences of the world are perceived as inseparable. Nurses

TABLE 5–1   THE FIVE PHASES OF NURSOLOGY.
1. Preparation of the nurse knower for coming to know
2. Nurse knowing of the other intuitively
3. Nurses knowing the other scientifically
4. Nurse complementarily synthesizing known others
5. Succession within the nurse from the many to the paradoxical one

(Patterson & Zderad, 1988)

who apply this method, consciously view the clinical experience as a *lived dialogue* between nurse and patient in the here and now. Using this technique, they see themselves and others as distinct human beings meeting at given points in time to engage in therapeutic relationships. The resulting dialogue extends beyond verbal and nonverbal communication, taking into account the whole of the present experience including intuition, feelings, and other perceptions.

The process has assumed the nomenclature of *phenomenologic nursology* which involves five phases that use reflection as a tool to examine the nurse and patient response to it (see Table 5–1). As a methodological starting point, Paterson and Zderad (1988) question the ways in which nurses have the capacity both subjectively and objectively to know themselves and their patients in the relationship. Before engaging in the activity, practitioners consider the individual's *angular view* and his or her *prereflective experience*.

The angular view indicates the person's unique vision of reality influenced by a particular outlook proclaimed at the time of an encounter. During the prereflective experience, a primary awareness exists, but its meaning has not yet been fully absorbed. The level of cognizance has an impact on both aspects of the person's perceptions regarding traumatic experiences and whether these experiences have been integrated and healed. As previously mentioned, trauma victims may see the world and others as unsafe until their hurt becomes conscious and integrated. Ipso facto, the nurse's viewpoint and ability to reflect will depend on the extent of healing that has taken place by the time of the encounter.

Preparation of the Nurse Knower for Coming to Know

This first phase requires an openness to experience what many people hesitate to embrace. At the outset, a necessary move involves preparing the mind to shift to higher levels of consciousness through activities without any direct relation to nursing. For example, consider reflecting on the humanities such as literature, poetry, music, and art and discuss their relevance to nurses and nursing practice. These creative modes of expression generate a multitude of ways to help individuals develop a broader perspective on the human condition. In this light, trauma survivors need to convert their perceptions to a larger and more recovery-oriented worldview. The humanities reveal not only the trials and tribulations of others, but the ways in which environmental obstacles can be surmounted.

Knowing of the Other Intuitively

In the second phase, nurses respond to the patient's uniqueness without personal judgment, being prepared for "surprise and question because the manner in which healing appears is often unanticipated for both nurse and patient" (Paterson & Zderad, 1988, p. 72). A prerequisite for intuitive knowing of the other begins with the "I," and with nurses it implies a capability for maintaining distance from the patient while still being present. Understanding the totality of the nurse-patient relationship occurs through the phenomenon of "I-thou-it-all-at-once," characterized by *being there*, a physical and psychological form of presence, which happens only when nurses accept themselves and focus completely on their patient's needs (Stiles, 1997).

Intuitive ability has always been identified with nursing practice and can be cultivated within the reflective process. Benner and Tanner (1987) refer to skilled pattern recognition, denoting that previously acquired knowledge and expertise represents the basis of intuition.

Knowing the Other Scientifically

Knowing the other scientifically will emerge after nurses understand the patient intuitively and the care required. This outcome depends on their view of the relationship and on how they synthesize themes or patterns and then interpret the essence of the human interaction. In this way as Buber (1965) proposes, knowledge is gathered and created through the knowing "I" transcending itself, recollecting, reflecting on, and experiencing the relationship as "I-it," with "it" being the nurse-patient relationship. The reflective state becomes a utilitarian as well as an extremely beneficial process for nurses as they analyze themselves vis-à-vis their clinical practice.

Nurse Complementarily Synthesizing Known Others

In this phase, nurses compare, contrast, and synthesize similarities and differences occurring in nursing situations designed to generate an expanded view. They examine and apply other concepts derived from developmental, psychological, and physiological theories, or perhaps from literature and art. The proposition of Johns (1995) that reflective practice focuses on the contradictions in practice should be considered since questions may arise about how nursing is actually performed.

Succession within the Nurse from the Many to the Paradoxical One

This final phase depicts the nurse creating a fresh perspective on a particular situation and acquiring greater understanding. The "many" refers to the multiplicity of interpretations offered, even though a paradox may appear in the conclusion arrived at by the nurse. For example, he or she may believe through experience and an intuitive leap that a seriously ill patient wishes to live although verbalizing the will to die. At this juncture, personal insight as well as knowledge of the clinical situation becomes critical, enabling practitioners to apply what they have already learned in their practice. Carefully thought out, a pattern reflecting growth follows with a changing view and alternatives created to improve responses to patient care.

THE SEARCH WITHIN

Lumby (1998) focuses her work on reflective practice within the context of a search for meaning and its transformational potential for nurses. She cites the following four phases in the process: (1) searching for meaning, (2) making meaning, (3) transforming meaning, and (4) sharing meaning.

Searching for Meaning

As in nursology, searching for meaning requires an analysis of the nurse-patient dialogue by both participants. A variety of methods can be employed such as making tape recordings, maintaining a journal of personal observations, and questioning and note taking. During the interaction, levels of meaning begin to emerge from the interpersonal exchange. In addition to the more formalized documentation of experience, "incidental reflections" may surface during informal telephone conversations but the content tends to be more superficial. On later examination, reflective materials can be exchanged so that each participant contemplates the other's revelations.

Making Meaning

In what Lumby (1998) portrays as an emotionally difficult phase known as critical conversation, the nurse and patient assess their interactions and attempt to understand the meaning of each other's perceptions. Whether productive or otherwise, the results will depend largely on the nurse's veracity in the dialogue. The patient also may find it difficult to face the issues detected, especially if the significance of the health problem surfaces. For example, in the case of a middle-aged smoker who became addicted during the teenage years, the behavior may have become a dysfunctional way of avoiding emotional problems. During the nurse-patient analysis, the participants may determine that smoking provided symbolic protection from an inner fear of vulnerability. On further examination, however, specific behaviors can evolve that may help the patient understand the root of the problem and its impact on his or her life.

Transforming Meaning

During this phase, narratives acquired from the interactive process can be compiled with the aim of producing significant themes. Often, a compelling personal transformation and transcendence for both individuals occur as a result of studying the material. Lumby (1998) states that these transformative techniques can also be useful in focus groups of practitioners or students, formed to uncover information and to assist them in moving through levels of reflection. Descriptive diaries and recordings of dialogue allow practitioners to distance themselves from traumatic material. The results may produce an increased awareness of several perspectives that ultimately transform the affected individuals.

Sharing Meaning

In the final stage, theory and practice become inseparable as the participants incorporate the changes resulting from their shared experiences into consciousness (Lumby, 1998). When transformation has been integrated into awareness, one can never again be the same, and growth based on the new behavior patterns assumes enormous potential. Sharing transformation narratives also makes the lived experience of change more real for the person and others, providing rich material for further insight and growth. Such storytelling engenders hope as nurses become effective role models for sharing buried feelings and traumatic experiences in their effort to transform themselves.

INTEGRATION OF TRAUMA

The integrative approach to reaching resolution with a search for meaning requires not only reflection but the synthesis of cognitive and emotional residuals of the trauma. van der Kolk (2000) suggests that the memories of wounded individuals may be more somatic than semantic because sensory elements of the traumatic episode often remain separately lodged in the brain and surface later on in life, without words to describe them. As Levine and Frederick (1997) point out, the emotions become frozen through body memories without being easily released through verbal therapies or traditional left brain functions, such as speech or cognitive thought. Interpreting meaning alone may not be enough to heal traumatic experiences; it therefore becomes an important reminder for wounded professionals, whose own trauma may be covertly triggered by the clinical setting.

According to some authorities, trauma therapy aims to help individuals transcend their reactions to past feelings, to live fully in the present, and to respond to their circumstances with greater ease (van der Kolk, McFarlane, & van der Hart, 1996). Treatment entails three critical steps that include ensuring safety, anxiety management, and emotional processing.

Ensuring safety must be stressed because wounded individuals require new experiences that contradict the emotional and often physical helplessness emanating from a traumatic event. Positive support from family, friends, therapists, and perhaps colleagues can offset the fears they experience. During this phase, patients may need extensive education regarding the nature and dynamics of their wounding so as to begin building anew a framework for changing their view of the world as an unsafe place. They also may be asked to explore their emotional and physical responses in a trusting environment, exposing them openly and decreasing the sense of isolation. The process can be especially helpful in showing the incongruity between past emotions and present circumstances.

Another step, that of managing anxiety, may emerge in the form of relaxation, meditation, breath control, role playing, guided imagery, and specific types of body work if the patient can tolerate it. Antianxiety medications can also play a role in treatment when the individual's arousal level does not decrease easily. In addition, identifying problems and formulating appropriate solutions are part of this phase (van der Kolk, 2000). Modulating anxious arousal may be the most important feature of integration because it enables the person to cope more effectively and assimilate the traumatic material when in a calm state.

Finally, emotional processing requires a reexperiencing of the trauma without the person's feeling helpless. Various forms of *exposure therapy* promote symptom alleviation by allowing patients to realize that remembering a trauma does not mean it exists in the present but that it has been part of their history (van der Kolk, 2000). Although one popular behaviorist technique called "systematic desensitization" exposes the patient to the feared stimulus while in a state of complete relaxation so as to decrease arousal levels, it has produced only mixed results relieving anxiety (Olasov, Rothbaum, & Foa, 1996).

Another method, known as "eye movement desensitization and reprocessing" (EMDR®) has been reported as having more success. During the procedure, the patient is asked to maintain an image of the original traumatic episode and to focus on the feelings and physiological arousal associated with it while tracking the practitioner's rapidly moving finger. As the technique progresses, the eye movements tend to exacerbate troubling memories, until the sequence is repeated and the patient no longer reports anxiety (Parnell, 1997).

EMDR operates on the premise that inducing rapid eye movement (REM) in a wakeful state helps heal the wounded individual naturally through a process similar to that of dreaming. Theoretically, trauma can be resolved through dreams, yet frightening content may awaken the wounded individual and interrupt the process. By simulating a REM, the practitioner maintains the patient's eyes in motion and helps the patient focus on the occurrence, allowing it to be fully experienced and processed (Parnell, 1997). Marked circumspection is essential in performing the procedure since the patient may be flooded with extremely painful memories. If unable to cope, increased awareness of traumatic memories can occur with associated negative feelings such as shame and guilt and self-destructive behaviors (van der Kolk, 2000).

The following scenario shows how a 32-year-old nurse with a master's degree partially integrated her traumatic past, which heightened her awareness of certain dysfunctional patterns. Nevertheless, she continued to remain despondent because she did not fully understand the meaning of her wounding.

Before assuming her present position in public health administration, Kelly worked for five years in a medical intensive-care unit. Her background revealed a family history with an alcoholic father and a depressed, code-pendent, mother. She described herself as the "parenting child," the oldest of seven siblings. Since many of the families in her community abused alcohol, Kelly might be perceived as having grown up in an alcoholic culture. She remembered clearly her childhood trips to the local bar after school to bring her inebriated father home, an activity that was commonplace to many children in the neighborhood. Conscious at an early age of the effects of ongoing familial trauma, particularly emotional abandonment, she attempted to counteract her feelings of helplessness by assuming control through the parenting of her siblings.

In adopting this role, Kelly developed confidence in her judgment and projected an authoritative voice. In time, she adopted a pattern of "public defender" to compensate for the trauma of parental neglect and rejection. By supporting and rescuing other dysfunctional people, she could then avoid the shame of being part of an alcoholic family. Her situation, however, created a psychological isolation because she focused on others in a pattern of oversolicitude and neglected to develop goals of her own. As a teenager, she exhibited symptoms of overwork, overexercising, and bulimia all of which persisted.

During her preparation as a nursing student, an incident on a clinical unit mirrored Kelly's early childhood experience when she was assigned to care for Bridget, a young woman being treated for alcohol addiction. The patient also suffered from a severe case of bulimia which had not been addressed by the other staff. Bridget informed the student of her bingeing and purging while in treatment and indicated that no one had listened to or recognized her needs.

Kelly identified immediately with the patient particularly because of the eating disorder and the feelings of frustration that endured over the years, which had gone undetected by those around her. Reflecting on the problem, she immediately recognized her own trauma pattern related to the roles of parent and public defender and persuaded the health care team on the unit to explore Bridget's problem more deeply. Although she was able to pursue a healthy outcome for the patient, the pattern arising from her own personal wounding was not altered.

Kelly had not dealt with the basis of her wounding up to that time but she could identify the symptoms that produced certain patterns in her life. Eventually, however, the reenactment with Bridget had a positive effect because it increased her insight and motivated her to seek therapy for the source of the problems that had remained deeply embedded and unresolved.

SUMMARY

Reflection, which evolved out of introspective theory practiced throughout the decades, represents a valuable tool in the journey toward healing that precedes the important process of trauma integration. Through reflection-in-action and reflection-on-action, practitioners can examine themselves from both personal and professional perspectives.

Biblical and mythological references from ancient times illustrate reflection as a way of scrutinizing repetitive dysfunctional patterns as well as a means of confronting and overcoming them. In the process known as phenomenologic nursology, practitioners and their patients grow together, with the nurse illuminating the situation and fostering greater understanding. In the context of searching for meaning and the transformational potential, several methods can be used to analyze the dialogue.

Discarding the wounded inner child identity requires sacrificing patterns that inhibit self-awareness, such as excessive talking, expressing negative emotions, excessive fantasy, and clinging to suffering. The process of integrating trauma through reflective practice assumes the entirety of the individual's experience that includes intuition, feeling, and various perceptions.

DISCUSSION GUIDE

1. Discuss the differences between reflection-in-action and reflection-on-action.
2. Analyze the stories of the raven, Perseus, and Lot's wife and their relationship to the wounded healer.
3. Describe the practice of self-talk and how it relates to mental health.
4. Explain how the search for meaning helps trauma resolution.
5. What is the significance of trauma integration, and cite some techniques for achieving it?

REFERENCES

Bailey, J. (1998). The supervisor's story: From expert to novice. In C. Johns & D. Freshwater (Eds.), *Transforming nursing through reflective practice* (pp. 194–205). London: Blackwell Science.

Benner, P. (1984). *From novice to expert: Excellence and power in clinical nursing practice.* Menlo Park, CA: Addison-Wesley.

Benner, P., & Tanner, C. (1987). How expert nurses use intuition. *American Journal of Nursing, 1,* 23–31.

Bepko, C., & Krestan, J. A. (1985). *The responsibility trap: A blueprint for treating the alcoholic family.* New York: Free Press.

Buber, M. (1965). *Between man and man* (R. G. Smith, Trans.). New York: Macmillan. (Original work published 1937)

Carroll, L. *Alice's adventures in Wonderland.* New York: Knopf.

Early, E. (1993). *The raven's return: The influence of psychological trauma on individuals and culture.* Wilmette, IL: Chiron.

Ellis, A., & Harper, R. (1975). *A new guide to rational living.* North Hollywood, CA: Wilshire.

James W. (1950). *The principles of psychology* (Vols.1–2). New York: Kover.

Johns, C. (1995). The value of reflective practice for nursing. *Journal of Clinical Nursing, 4,* 23–30.

Johns, C., & Freshwater, D. (Eds.). (1998). *Transforming nursing through reflective practice.* London: Blackwell Science.

Levine, P., & Frederick, A. (1997). *Walking the tiger: Healing trauma.* Berkeley, CA: North Atlantic.

Lumby, J. (1998). Transforming nursing through reflective practice. In C. Johns & D. Freshwater (Eds.), *Transforming nursing through reflective practice.* (pp. 91–103). London: Blackwell Science.

Olasov-Rothbaum, B., & Foa, E. B. (1996). Cognitive-behavioral therapy for posttraumatic stress disorder. In B. van der Kolk, A.C. McFarlane, & L. Weisaeth (Eds.), *Traumatic stress: The effects of overwhelming experience on mind, body and society* (pp. 491–509). New York: Guilford.

Ouspensky, P. D. (1981). *The psychology of man's possible evolution.* New York: Vintage.

Parnell, L. (1997). *Transforming trauma: EMDR®: The revolutionary new therapy for freeing the mind, clearing the body and opening the heart.* New York: Norton.

Patterson, J. G., & Zderad, L. T. (1988). *Humanistic nursing.* New York: NLN.

Pinkola-Estes, C. (1992). *Women who run with wolves: Myths and stories of the wild woman archetype.* New York: Ballantine.

Rutter, P. (1995). Lot's wife, Sabina Spielrein and Anita Hill: A Jungian meditation on sexual boundary abuse and recovery of lost voices. In J. C. Gonsiorek (Ed.), *Breach of trust: Sexual exploitation by health care professionals and clergy* (pp. 75–80). Thousand Oaks, CA: Sage.

Schön, D. (1983). *The reflective practitioner: How professionals think in action.* New York: Basic Books.

Stiles, K. A. (1997). Being there: The healing power of presence. *Alternative and Complementary Therapies, 4,* 133–139.

Taylor, B. (1998). Locating a phenomenological perspective of reflective nursing and midwifery practice by contrasting interpretive and critical reflection. In C. Johns & D. Freshwater (Eds.), *Transforming nursing through reflective practice* (pp. 134–150). London: Blackwell Science.

Titchener, E. B. (1912). The schema of introspection. *American Journal of Psychology, 23,* 485–508.

van der Kolk, B., (2000). The assessment and treatment of complex PTSD. In R. Yehuda (Ed.), *Traumatic stress* (pp. 1–20). Washington, DC: American Psychiatric Press.

van der Kolk, B. McFarlane, A. C., & van der Hart, O. (1996). A general approach to treatment of posttraumatic stress disorder. In B. van der Kolk, A. C. McFarlane, & L. Weisaeth (Eds.), *Traumatic stress: The effects of overwhelming experience on mind, body and society* (pp. 417–440). New York: Guilford.

Willis, P. (1999). Looking for what it's really like: Phenomenology in reflective practice. *Studies in Continuing Education, 21* (10), 91–112.

Wolinsky, S. (1993). *The dark side of the inner child: The next step.* Fall Village, CT: Bramble.

Woodman, M. (1990). *Addiction to perfection: The roots of compulsive behavior and the need for spiritual fulfillment.* [Audiocassette] Boston: Shambhala.

Wundt, W. (1897). *Outlines of psychology.* Leipzig, Germany: Engelmann.

CHAPTER 6

JOURNEY'S END: TRANSFORMATION AND TRANSCENDENCE

Seed of the blood of gods, Trojan son of Anchises, the descent to Hades is easy. All day and all night the portal of Dis is open: but to retrace your steps and escape to the air above, this is the problem and this the task.

Virgil, *The Aeneid*

After examining the nature and effect of a traumatic event, the ultimate step in the journey of the wounded healer involves transformation and transcendence. Through the process of transforming, we can alter the character, substance, or function of an entity by restructuring what has existed (Wade, 1998). Another view is that a metamorphosis may occur, literally meaning a change of form.

Transformation can be likened to the odyssey of the butterfly, whose basic essence remains constant during its transfiguration from caterpillar to isolative cocoon and finally to its emergence as a beautifully colored air-borne creature. In human terms, the struggle to become a "new" person may be traumatic and even fraught with danger as the individual moves through various stages of development. As the butterfly transforms, remarkable possibilities ensue through the capability of flight. So too, when nurses strive toward becoming wounded healers, they often encounter adversity along the way but at the same time acquire greater levels of depth and healing potential for themselves and others. Myss (1997) refers to illness as the "transformative vehicle" because it allows us to develop into more whole human beings by opening our eyes, gaining different perspectives about life, and perhaps helping to transcend the present (p. 101).

Personal transformation represents a dynamic, uniquely individualized force, expanding consciousness and allowing the person to become vitally aware of existing and newer self-perceptions, and then choosing to integrate them into a revised self-definition (Wade, 1998). Newman (1988) points out that when we expand consciousness, our action moves us toward transformation by generating insight into patterns of behavior after synthesizing contradictory events or disturbances in the flow of everyday life. She asserts that transformation begins with the person, which implies discarding certain

87

preconceived notions. By believing in the good of a Higher Level of Consciousness, we can accept ourselves, encourage such emotions as love, and allow change to occur. Underlying this premise evolves a theory of transpersonal consciousness that perceives the universe as a dynamic web of relationships in a state of continual change (Vaughn, 1979).

Transformation and transcendence may be viewed as two sides of the same coin, characterized by an interdependence and allowing the individual to go beyond what exists so as to achieve a new level of growth. In this light, the more compelling question to be addressed is "What am I transcending and how does it happen?" The key to the process comes with the recognition of transforming from the walking wounded into wounded healer by transcending past and present circumstances.

Karen, a 35-year-old school nurse, illustrates the above observation. When assuming her present position four years earlier, she had no conscious understanding of her motivation for selecting this field of nursing, which was largely due to her inability to bear children. She had rationalized this career choice by citing the shorter work hours and the proximity of the school to her home. According to her employment history, she had worked previously in an acute care setting and during that period, underwent several expensive and unsuccessful treatments for infertility which created marked feelings of failure.

Subsequently, after six years in acute care, Karen decided to switch to school nursing. However, almost from the outset she began to experience little job satisfaction. Before long, she found that working with children did not meet her expectations, because of a continuing desire for a family of her own. Her conflicting interests prompted her to self-examine in greater depth, and eventually she became aware of the disappointment she harbored within herself. Acquiring further insights, she transformed her situation into one of self-acceptance rather than self-recrimination and decided to return to an adult care setting.

Adams (1986) believes that transformation emerges from fundamental changes in thought and action that cause dissonance in the individual's experience. In essence, persons can no longer be comfortable with prior behavior and thought patterns. As a result, they adopt new belief systems radically different from the previous ones and alter their behavior. Therefore, once awareness comes to the surface, past practices disappear.

MOVING TOWARD TRANSCENDENCE

Maslow (1969), a pioneer in humanistic psychology, has offered a compendium of interpretations relating to transcendence. Among 35 meanings, he highlights one definition that describes the process in which the individual applies his or her own past as a prerequisite for healing. In this regard, previous happenings can be embraced and fully accepted with forgiveness and understanding, while simultaneously relinquishing remorse, regret, guilt, shame, embarrassment, and other self-deprecating feelings. To achieve this level of transcendence, the highest, most inclusive, and holistic human consciousness needs to be attained.

Maslow's (1969) observations differ markedly from viewing past circumstances in relation to helplessness, because some personal responsibility must be assumed for the past: one cannot simply blame the situation on outside forces. He equates transcendence with the "peak experience," a manifestation of self-actualization. Since individuals can have many such experiences, the potential for transcendence is limitless.

An outstanding example of transcendence can be found in the life of Viktor Frankl, a German-born psychiatrist and Holocaust survivor. As a concentration camp inmate, he concluded that people who survived the horrendous existence in the camps had discovered meaning in their sufferings because of a powerful need to live for the sake of their loved ones. He also believed that the camps themselves symbolized the capacity for self-transcendence, pointing out that although man invented the gas chambers of Auschwitz, there were people who went to their deaths walking upright with prayers on their lips (Scully, 1995). Later Frankl (1966) claimed self-transcendence to be the core of existence, with self-actualization as only a side effect.

Transcendence and healing are desirable goals for nurses and their patients, with the level attained by both participants determining the therapeutic nature of the relationship. Zukav (1989) contends that healing may or may not occur in the mutual interaction, depending on "whether the personality involved can see beyond itself and that of the other personality to the interaction of their souls, an act that automatically brings forth compassion" (p. 42). Upchurch (1999) corroborates this belief in that individuals develop over the course of a lifetime by making personal choices within the context of their environment. The greater authenticity revealed in their selections, the healthier the result. Because the nature of personal essence has been so intimately involved with recovery, transcendence of a trauma's aftereffect must take place before healing can be engendered in others.

Theoretical Interpretations in Nursing

Watson (1988) reminds us that human beings transcend nature while continuing to remain a part of it. In this way, a model exists for understanding transcendence in which it is possible to observe and be the observed at the same time. We can view ourselves through the medium of consciousness—past, present, and future—perceiving our state of health and healing potential. Past wounds may be recalled and transcended through self-examination, and this process to a great extent determines the direction of our lives.

Within the nurse-patient dyad, each participant enters into what Watson (1988) terms "a transpersonal caring relationship where a spiritual union occurs between the two persons, both capable of transcending self, time, and space and the life history of the other" (p. 67). Therefore, both become part of one another's domain, creating a larger and more complex healing experience. Watson's (1988) theory brings nursing into the metaphysical realm and into a deeper level of abstraction where a higher sense of wholeness exists and the soul and transcendence are incorporated.

Martha Rogers (1990) has based much of her work on the concepts of transcendence and self-transcendence, in which the former appears as an evolutionary process, an inherent characteristic of the human environmental energy field. In particular, the Rogerian principle of *helicy*, "the continuous, innovative, unpredictable increasing diversity of human and environmental field patterns," epitomizes transformation and transcendence (Rogers, 1992, p. 31). From her discourse, we see the nurse, patient, and environment as inseparable in an upward spiral of growth, which can be hastened by increasingly higher levels of consciousness.

Commenting on the state of nursing science in the space age, Rogers (1992) explains that "humankind is on the threshold of a new cosmology, transcending an earthbound past" (p. 24). Nurses and patients transcend themselves, their situations, and perhaps eventually, their earthly realms. Reed's (1991a) theory of self-transcendence builds on Rogerian concepts, including the precept of "pandimensional" awareness, which extends beyond the physical body and time and occurs in patterns of increasing complexity and organization.

In Newman's (1990) view, nurses foster transcendence when they help patients expand consciousness and acquire a fuller understanding of the health patterns needed to generate change. Transcendence involves caring, pattern recognition, and movement toward greater complexity and creativity encompassing an inner reality that depicts the reality of the whole person (Reed, 1996). Barrett (1988) suggested earlier that nurses and patients deliberately and voluntarily work toward transforming and transcending patterns of illness to achieve better health.

Parse (1987) describes the process of mobilizing transcendence as one that moves beyond the "meaning moment" which has not yet happened and that occurs by dreaming of what is possible and planning to fulfill it. Since the nurse and patient are inseparable, they cotranscend the possibilities for change after exploring the meanings that exist in the present situation. Parse (1992) accentuates the necessity of cotranscending endless possibilities as a major impetus for reaching transformation and transcendence, whereas Leppanen-Montgomery (1996) sees transcendence as experiencing oneself as a part of a greater force within the nurse-patient relationship.

Achieving Self-Transcendence

Self-transcendence as interpreted by Reed (1991a) is based on her research with older adults. It has also been studied in women with breast cancer (Coward, 1991) and patients infected with the human immunodeficiency virus (Mellors, Riley, & Erlen, 1997). Concurring with Erikson (1986), Reed (1991b) contends that the process follows a developmental course, in which individuals as they mature become less focused on personal interests and more on their desire to be needed. She defines the experience of the individual as reaching inwardly through introspection or reflection, outwardly with concern for others, and temporally by means of perceptions of the past and future that enhance the present.

In the process of transcending, personal boundaries may be perceived as open and extending beyond immediate or constricted views and thus become more oriented toward external perspectives, activities, and purposes. Negating the person's value should be avoided, since examining the more unflattering aspects of one's personality and life may be resisted even when potential exists for transformation and growth. As shown in Margaret's story that follows, healing for the nurse and patient may require exploring negative patterns that contribute initially to illness too painful to endure.

Margaret, a 25-year-old woman with a bachelor's degree in nursing, had worked on a surgical nursing unit since obtaining her licensure. The family history revealed her mother to be a compulsive overeater and her father chemically dependent. As a child, she developed the same eating disorder as her mother and resorted to extensive overexercising. The pattern continued into adulthood when she still could not control her weight, experiencing feelings of anger and frustration.

Finally, Margaret sought a professional therapist and began to understand that her overeating had become a major impediment to her own self-awareness and resulted in wasted energy and addictive behaviors. She decided to study holistic nursing and worked in a clinic where AMMA therapy was used to treat patients. By then, she had lost weight, changed her eating patterns, and believed that she had transcended much of the negativity learned in childhood.

Margaret's emotional growth became apparent one day when she had an opportunity to treat Lisa, a 22-year-old clinic patient, who was complaining of unrelieved shoulder pain and fatigue. During the session, which was the young woman's first exposure to body work, Lisa casually mentioned having a weight problem as a college student that had greatly upset her. Because of her own overweight history, Margaret could relate easily to the young woman and suspected that her physical symptoms and fatigue could be traced to the anger stemming from Lisa's eating disorder.

In preparing for the treatment, the nurse centered herself and reflected on the principles of Traditional Chinese Medicine, which attributes the major cause of all illness to the emotions. She believed that Lisa's pain represented a blockage of energy (Qi) related to a pattern of stagnant liver functioning caused by the patient's anger.

During the encounter, Margaret massaged the patient's neck and shoulders to promote relaxation. She also manipulated the liver channel located on the front of the body, and applied the proper pressure. Much of the treatment was nonverbal, but when it ended, Lisa declared that her pain had disappeared and that she had not expected the experience to be so powerful. She began to reveal in some detail, and with a marked release of anger, her hidden problem with bulimia. Lisa thanked Margaret profusely for helping her not only physically but for making it possible for her to understand her addictive behavior and its consequences.

Symbols, Metaphors, and Myths

In addition to theory and language, the complex processes of transformation and transcendence can often be better understood through the application of symbols, metaphors, and stories. As an ancient and fundamental instrument of knowledge, symbolism reveals aspects of reality that escape other modes of expression (Cooper, 1978, p. 7). It transcends cultural and generational forces that may lead to more immediate explication of meaning. In this light, the caduceus has been mentioned as a symbol of transformation and rebirth. It should be noted, however, that in the case of shamans, the existence of the wound may be the most important symbol in interpreting the meaning of the wounded healer.

By communicating meaning, imagery can suggest paths for action or practice (Smith, 1992). Its use has a way of transferring something complex and often unknown in an instantaneous flash (Watson, 1987). In the title of his autobiography, Audie Murphy (1988), an American military hero of World War II, used the metaphor of going "to hell and back" to describe the nature of combat. The work gives a graphic portrayal of the nature of war through images of fighting demons, suffering, and becoming wounded. His experience may also figuratively describe the journey of the wounded healer.

Of interest is that ancient mythology often alludes to descending into hell or the underworld prior to transcendence. In modern times, this painful occurrence has been referred to as "the dark night of the soul" during which individuals come to know themselves more fully by confronting fears and formerly held beliefs, allowing them to experience, comprehend, and accept the *Shadow* nature (Myss, 1996).

Myths represent stories that incorporate symbols and metaphors to enhance our understanding of human phenomena. They can help or hinder the process of growth, depending on their interpretations and view of truth to explain reality. Furthermore, they help clarify abstract concepts as well as common everyday happenings. Unfortunately, they can also impede us when we cling too strongly to them instead of taking risks to move toward growth.

According to Campbell (1990), myths focusing on heroes or heroines follow the same pattern in most cultures where the protagonist departs from the ordinary world, descends into the underworld confronting both hostile and helpful forces, and transcends a serious challenge while gaining a worthy reward. Through transformation of the experience, an expansion of consciousness results as well as significant change.

Symbols in the Wounded Healer's Journey

In classical mythology, the cave, the underworld, and the quest illustrate the processes of transformation and transcendence, with many of the elements present in the wounded healer archetype. In addition to being the symbol of the universe as well as the world center or place of union for the self and the ego, the cave also has symbolic relevance in a number of cultures. As noted earlier, the Chinese view the cave as the feminine *yin* whereas the opposite is the mountain, or masculine *yang*. Yet, the cave exists within the mountain and vice versa, reflecting their interdependence (Cooper, 1978). It has also become a major symbol with the activities surrounding it serving as metaphors for change.

In another interpretation, the cave is perceived as the portal to the unconscious and the path to forces that contribute to our development as human beings (Crisp, 1990). Recall the case of Chiron, the wounded healer, who retreated to his cave where he worked in solitude after sustaining his injury. The act of passing through the entrance implies the beginning of a transformational process (Cooper, 1978). Many important experiences occur in caves that serve as meeting places for the mortal and the divine. There, gods die and saviors are born, acquiring esoteric knowledge during their lifetimes. Even temporarily, it sometimes becomes necessary to spend time away from the outside world to gain some enlightenment.

Virgil, the Roman poet, characterized part of the underworld as a place reserved for mortals, who through their virtuous lives earned a blessed afterlife. These are the Elysian Fields, or Elysium, a paradise for its inhabitants to live a purer, more carefree, and pleasant existence (Wilson, 2000). In psychological terms, the underworld typifies the hidden side of the self, similar to the Jungian concept of the *Shadow*.

Reed (1996) suggests that in Plato's *Republic* (1949), the cave is viewed allegorically as illuminating the processes affecting transformation and transcendence. In the story, cave dwellers lived in an underground den with an opening facing the light and extending along the entire area. Restrained since childhood, they were unable to move with their legs and necks chained. In such circumstances, they could not see the light, only what appeared in front of them, including the shadows cast on the wall by the firelight.

The cave dwellers believed the shadows to be authentic because they lacked knowledge of any external forces. According to Socrates, if any of the inhabitants were to exit from the cave, they would have difficulty returning after discovering that life inside was an illusion (Heuerman & Olson, 2000). Furthermore, any attempt to inform the remaining cave dwellers that their lives were based on a fallacy could have deleterious consequences. Those who achieved transcendence would be viewed as threatening and as potential sources of danger rather than wisdom, and the internal cave dwellers might hold on more firmly to their previous beliefs.

Plato's story of the cave clearly shows the deceptive world of appearances, whereas the outside journey reflects the ascent to knowledge (Heuerman & Olson, 2000). Thus, it would appear that people trapped by illusions have limited understanding of reality. By making a concerted effort, however, they have the capability to free themselves from erroneous perceptions and expand consciousness to a higher realm.

Journeys into caves often precede forays into the underworld, which in many cultural myths represent the lowest level housing the spirits of the dead. Separated from the world of the living by an impassable abyss or river, only mortals with a divinelike nature can descend and transcend its borders. Unlike the Judeo-Christian concept of hell, symbolizing eternal damnation, the suffering in the underworld is more varied in nature. There, the dead endure a flavorless and unhappy existence, frequently drinking from Lethe, the "river of forgetfulness," prior to experiencing reincarnation (Parada, 1997). This outcome gives credence to the notion that transformation requires letting go of the past and seeking a readiness to find a new life.

The stories of Aeneas, Jason, and the quest for the Holy Grail demonstrate the relevance of the cave, the quest, and the underworld to the process of transforming and transcending (Parada, 1997). Credited with the founding of Rome, Aeneas was born from the union of the mortal, Anchises, and the goddess Aphrodite. When wounded during the Trojan War, his rescuer Apollo, the divine physician, brought him to the temple at Pergamus to be healed. While recovering, Aeneas became even stronger than before and returned victoriously to the battlefield.

With the fall of Troy, he left the burning city to sail the Mediterranean, reaching Italy and approaching the entrance to the underworld. Upon receiving approval from the gods to visit his deceased father, he entered the cave and saw grief, anxiety, diseases, old age, fear, hunger, death, and agony. In the distant fields were the souls who died in childhood, and others who committed suicide as well as the unborn. Aeneas also observed some souls drinking from the waters of the river Oblivion before rebirth. He finally met with Anchises, who prophesied that his son would have a glorious future as the progenitor of the Roman civilization. Guided out of the underworld by his father, he was transformed by the experience and fulfilled his destiny by founding the Eternal City.

As another hero in Greek mythology, Jason traveled the path to becoming a wounded healer after encountering severe adversity. He was sent away for 20 years to be reared by Chiron when marital infidelity disgraced his family and his father lost the throne. Subsequently transformed, he emerged from Chiron's cave determined to restore his father to power.

To prevent Jason from fulfilling the mission, his uncle Pelias persuaded him to embark on a long voyage to remove the Golden Fleece, a revered and almost unattainable object from the horns of a dragon that never slept. Pelias hoped that the undertaking would result in Jason's death and eliminate any claim to the crown. During the perilous voyage, Jason and his companions the Argonauts encountered many trials, but he succeeded in his quest and saved his father's good name and throne (Parada, 1997).

The Mythic Quest to Transcendence

Since the mythic quest symbolizes the goal of achieving transformation and transcendence, it has relevance to the wounded healer as demonstrated by the search for the Holy Grail. Believed to have been the cup used by Jesus at the Last Supper and in which Joseph of Arimathea collected the blood flowing from Christ's side at the Crucifixion, it was brought to Britain and kept there for centuries ("Holy Grail," Microsoft® Encarta® Online Encyclopedia, 2000). The sacred object was thought to have been concealed in a mysterious castle surrounded by a wasteland and guarded by a custodian called the Fisher King, who suffered from a wound that would not heal. It was purported that the man had been struck mute at the sight of the Grail because of his sinful ways and that his recovery and the renewal of lands that had been laid to ruin depended upon the successful quest for the chalice.

Near the end of King Arthur's reign, Merlin the magician proclaimed that every knight of the Round Table must seek the sacred cup. Percival, a youth aspiring to join the elite group, embarked on the quest. Upon arriving at the Fisher King's castle, the boy witnessed an unusual procession where the Grail and the spear that pierced Christ's side (which was bleeding) were passed before the voiceless sovereign. Percival learned later that if he, a pure and guileless soul would have spoken out at the time, the Fisher King's wound would have been healed ("Percival," Microsoft® Encarta® Online Encyclopedia, 2000). After wandering in search of his true love and marrying her, he returned to the castle, restored the power of speech to the Fisher King, and then succeeded him. ("Arthurian Legend," Micrsoft® Encarta® Online Encyclopedia, 2000).

It can be speculated that Florence Nightingale had embarked on a mythic quest when she went to Kaiserwerth, and later Scutari. Perhaps her earlier visits to Egypt and Greece laid a foundation for an eventual personal transformation. Nightingale's spiritual journey reached a high level of intensity when she spent over three months on a Nile expedition and devoted much time to deep contemplation.

Montgomery-Dossey (2000) characterizes Nightingale as a mystic, an individual whose direct experience of God is transformed into a deeply personal experience. Nightingale's travels had deep personal meaning, comparable to a mystic's quest that entailed withdrawing from a familiar environment for the purpose of reevaluating previously held beliefs, goals, and values. Her journeys also seemed to have engendered such introspection, since after her excursion she commented, "I look back with pity and shame upon my former self, when I attached importance to my life and labors" (p. 63). As with mystics who entertain firm resolve to complete a new mission upon returning to their usual realms, Nightingale became ready to transform the world of nursing.

In Parthenope Nightingale's depiction of Florence after her quest, she is seen with a expression of determination. Interestingly, standing next to her is a small owl that she acquired in Greece. By naming the bird Athena after the goddess of wisdom, it seems to indicate that during her trip she underwent a process of profound transformation, from which a higher level of personal development emerged.

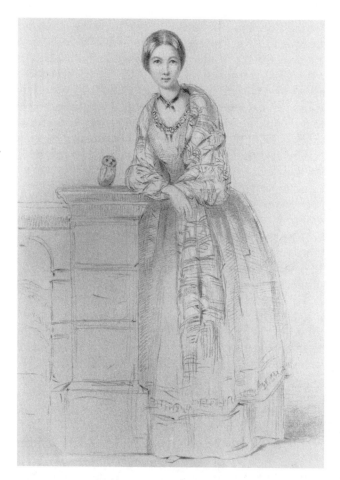

Figure 6–1 Florence Nightingale with Athena the owl, after a drawing by Parthenope Nightingale. With permission from the Florence Nightingale Museum, London.

Coming Apart: Coming Together

A legendary bird that lived in Arabia, the phoenix may be perceived as the ultimate and inspiring example of transformation and transcendence. According to tradition, it consumed itself by fire every 500 years and a new, young phoenix sprang from its ashes. In the mythology of ancient Egypt, it represented the sun, which died at night and was reborn in the morning. Early Christian tradition adopted the phoenix as a symbol of both immortality and resurrection (Cooper, 1978). Although interpretations vary, the symbolism clearly indicates that sometimes a violent dissolution of the old must occur to make way for a transformation to the new.

In moving toward transformation, the individual must experience trials in an extreme sense and literally "come apart" so as to be reconnected later. In ancient Egypt, the brothers of Osiris, god of the underworld and vegetation, dismembered him until his wife, Isis, searched the land for the body parts and eventually put him back together again (Hillegass, 1973). In some Egyptian texts, dispersing body parts has been compared to the scattering of grain in the fields. Osiris symbolizes transformation as well as the creative forces of nature and the imperishability of life.

The descent of the Sumerian Goddess Innana into the underworld embodied a comprehensive application of dissolution and rebirth (Perera, 1981). Entering the netherworld, she had to remove an article of clothing at each of the protective gates. After Innana finally arrived at the dark goddess Ereskegal's chambers, she was killed and hung on a peg, leaving her body to decay. When she failed to return, Enki, the god of water and wisdom created two entities to go to the underworld to search for her. Upon their arrival, Ereskegal, being the "dark goddess," was consumed by her own depression and pain, but when the messengers manifested empathy, her suffering was alleviated. Subsequently Innana's corpse was returned and revived.

Perera's (1981) analysis of the above story reminds us that to be transformed often involves destroying a person's former identity. During the transition, the dark goddess within seems to demand complete destruction of the old self. As a result, symptoms such as a powerful depression may surface. Instead of seeking an immediate cure for these feelings, they may be viewed as part of a grieving process for the former self.

Alex Grey's *Journey of the Wounded Healer* (see Figure 6–2) portrays the concept of coming apart and reconnecting during the processes of transformation and self-transcendence. The first panel shows a being trapped and descending into the underworld of the dead, while caught in the limitation of the physical body. In the second panel, there appears an explosion and dismemberment on all levels and a three-headed serpent (symbol of rebirth) facilitating the transformation. The wounded healer emerges in the last panel, ascending the crystal mountain of the higher self empowered with the responsibility of healing the future (Grey, 1990). As Jung (1946) has proposed, only an arbitrary separation between therapist and patient occurs, and when both undergo the process of transformation and transcendence, more complex levels of healing can take place.

Color facsimiles of Figures 6–2A, 6–2B, and 6–2C may be found at the end of this book.

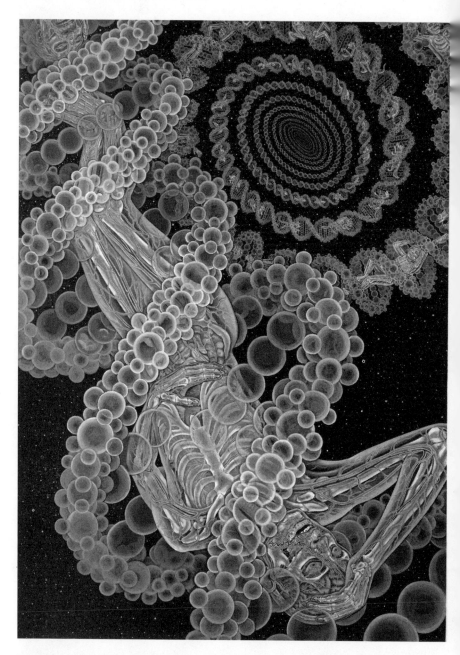

Figure 6–2A "Journey of the Wounded Healer," 1985, oil on linen, 216″ × 90″. From *Sacred Mirrors: The Visionary Art of Alex Grey*, Inner Traditions Publishing. In the collection of Museum of Contemporary Art, San Diego. (c)Alex Grey, *Journey of the Wounded Healer*. www.alexgrey.com

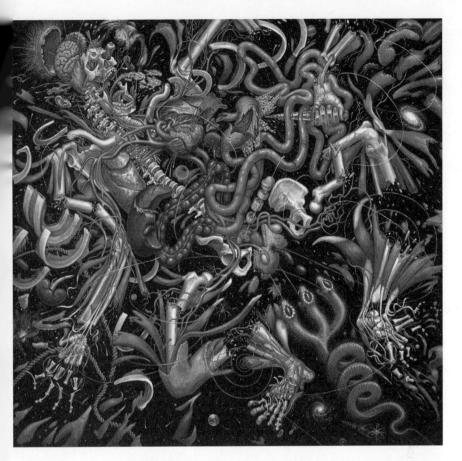

Figure 6–2B "Journey of the Wounded Healer," 1985, oil on linen, 216" × 90".
From *Sacred Mirrors: The Visionary Art of Alex Grey*, Inner Traditions Publishing. In the
collection of Museum of Contemporary Art, San Diego. (c)Alex Grey, *Journey of the
Wounded Healer*. www.alexgrey.com

SUMMARY

When the wounded healer reaches the stage of transformation, he or she will
have attained the desired goal of consciously understanding the nature of
the traumatic event. There evolves a critical awareness of present and new
self-perceptions integrated into a revised personal identity and reflecting
healthy change. Several nursing theorists offer illuminating interpretations of
the developmental course necessary to achieve transcendence. Symbols,
metaphors, and myths become significant accoutrements defining the
wounded healer's journey, in which destructive patterns followed by recon-
nection represent crucial components of the transformative process.

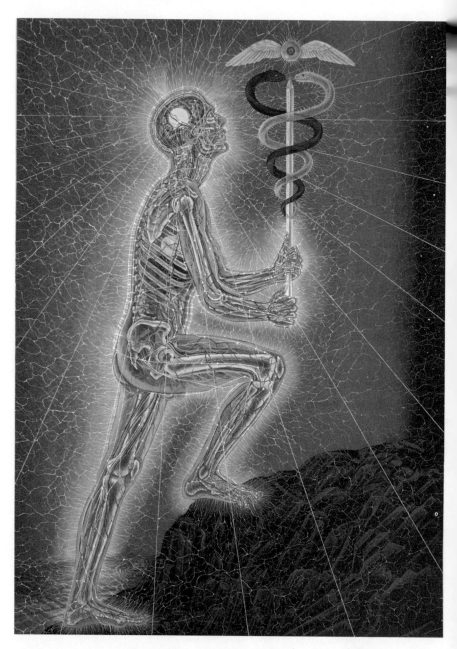

Figure 6–2C "Journey of the Wounded Healer," 1985, oil on linen, 216" × 90". From *Sacred Mirrors: The Visionary Art of Alex Grey*, Inner Traditions Publishing. In the collection of Museum of Contemporary Art, San Diego. (c)Alex Grey, *Journey of the Wounded Healer*. www.alexgrey.com

DISCUSSION GUIDE

1. Explore the differences between transformation, transcendence, and self-transcendence.
2. Identify some symbols and metaphors that have relevance in contemporary nursing practice.
3. Describe your interpretation of illness as a "transformative vehicle."
4. Explain Alex Grey's portrayal of the *Journey of the Wounded Healer* and its relevance to nursing.
5. Discuss Plato's allegory of the cave and the insights you derived from reading about it.

REFERENCES

Adams, J. D. (Ed.). (1986). *Transforming leadership: From vision to results.* Alexandria, VA: Miles River Press.

"Arthurian Legend" Microsoft® Encarta® Online Encyclopedia, 2000.

Barrett, E. A. M. (1988). Using Rogers' science of unitary human beings in nursing practice. *Nursing Science Quarterly,* 1, 50–51.

Campbell, J. (1990). *The hero with a thousand faces: Myths: Princeton Bollinger series in world mythology* (Vol. 17). Princeton, NJ: Princeton University Press.

Cooper, J. C. (1978). *An illustrated encyclopedia of traditional symbols.* London: Thames and Hudson.

Coward, D. (1991). Self-transcendency and emotional well-being in women with advanced breast cancer. *Oncology Nursing Forum,* 18, 162–169.

Crisp, T. (1990). *Dream dictionary.* New York: Dell.

Erikson, E. (1986). *Vital involvement in old age.* New York: Norton.

Frankl, V. (1966). Self-transcendence as a human phenomenon. *Journal of Humanistic Psychology,* 6, 97–106.

Grey, A. (1990). *Sacred mirrors: The visionary art of Alex Grey.* Rochester, VT: Inner Traditions International.

Heuerman, T., & Olson, J. (2000). The allegory of Plato's cave. *Self-Help and Psychology Magazine.* http.shpm.com.

Hillegass, C. K. (1973). *Cliff's notes on mythology.* Lincoln, NE: Cliffs Notes.

"Holy Grail," Microsoft® Encarta® Online Encyclopedia, 2000.

Jung, C. G. (1946). The psychology of transference. In H. Read, M. Fordham, G. Adler, & W. McGuire (Eds.), *The collected works of* C. G. Jung (CW 16). Princeton, NJ: Princeton University Press.

Leppanen-Montgomery, C. (1996). The care-giving relationship: Paradoxical and transcendent aspects. *Alternative Therapies,* 2 (2), 52–57.

Maslow, A. (1969). Various meanings of transcendence. *Journal of Transpersonal Psychology,* 1, 56–66.

Mellors, M., Riley, T., & Erlen, J. (1997). HIV, self-transcendence and quality of life. *Journal of the Association of Nurses in AIDS Care*, 8, 59–69.

Montgomery-Dossey, B. M. (2000). *Florence Nigthingale: Mystic, visionary, healer.* Springhouse, PA: Springhouse.

Murphy, A. (1988). *To hell and back.* Cutchogue, NY: Buccaneer. (Original work published in 1949).

Myss, C. (1996). *Anatomy of the spirit: The seven stages of power and healing.* New York: Three Rivers.

Myss, C. (1997). *Why people don't heal and how they can.* New York: Harmony.

Newman, M. (1988). *Health as expanding consciousness.* St. Louis: Mosby.

Newman, M. (1990). Shifting to higher consciousness. In M. E. Parker (Ed.), *Nursing theories in practice* (pp. 129–140). New York: NLN.

Parada, C. (1997). *Genealogical guide to Greek mythology.* Jonsered, Sweden: Astroms.

Parse, R. R. (1987). *Nursing science: Major paradigms, theories and critiques.* Philadelphia: Saunders.

Parse, R. R. (1992). Human becoming: Parse's theory of nursing. *Nursing Science Quarterly*, 5 35–42.

"Percival" Microsoft® Encarta® Online Encyclopedia, 2000.

Perera, S. B. (1981). *Descent to the goddess: A way of initiation for women.* Toronto: Inner City.

Plato. (1949). *Republic: Books VI–VII.* Chicago: Regnery.

Reed, P. (1991a). Toward a theory of self-transcendence: Deductive transformation using developmental theories. *Advances in Nursing Science*, 13, 64–77.

Reed, P. (1991b). Self-transcendence and mental health in oldest-old adults. *Nursing Research*, 40, 1–7.

Reed, P. (1996). Transcendence: Formulating nursing perspectives. *Nursing Science Quarterly*, 9 (1), 2–4.

Rogers, M. E. (1990). Nursing science of unitary, irreducible human beings: Update 1990. In E. A. M. Barrett (Ed.), *Visions of Rogers' science based nursing* (pp. 5–11). New York: NLN Press.

Rogers, M. E. (1992). Nursing science and the space age. *Nursing Science Quarterly*, 5 (1), 27–34.

Scully, M. (1995). Viktor Frankl at ninety: An interview. *First Things*, 4, 39–43.

Smith, M. C. (1992). Metaphor in nursing theory. *Nursing Science Quarterly*, 5 (2), 48–49.

Upchurch, S. (1999). Self transcendence and activities of daily living: The woman with the pink slippers. *Journal of Holistic Nursing*, 17 (3), 251–266.

Vaughn, F. E. (1979). Transpersonal dimensions of psychotherapy. *Re-Vision*, 2 (1), 26–29.

Wade, G. H. (1998). A concept analysis of personal transformation. *Journal of Advanced Nursing*, 28 (4), 713–719.

Watson, J. (1987). Nursing on the caring edge: Metaphorical vignettes. *Advances in Nursing Science*, 10 (1), 10–18.

Watson, J. (1988). *Nursing: Human science and human caring: A theory of nursing.* New York: NLN.

Wilson, A. (2000). *Aeneas: The underworld.* www.classicspage.com

Zukav, G. (1989). *The seat of the soul.* New York: Simon & Schuster.

PART II

WOUNDED HEALERS: FACT AND FICTION

The wounded healer's journey is characterized by a number of pervasive themes exemplified by personal trauma, the quest for meaning, isolation, the choosing of one's destiny, increasing consciousness, and reemerging transcended. This phenomenon has been portrayed in various literary works that provide rich material for reflective practice. We are fortunate in being privy to fascinating stories about people throughout the ages and to the different ways they have communicated with one another.

From both fictional and factual accounts, nurses can share vicariously the experiences of our heroes and heroines and learn how they have coped with joy, sorrow, despair, and other human emotions. The outcome of such an exploration can generate more profound insights within ourselves as well as professional growth. Such enlightenment will help guide us in approaching our patients, students, and colleagues with greater understanding and sensitivity.

CHAPTER 7

FICTIONAL PORTRAYALS OF THE WOUNDED HEALER

AYLA: *CLAN OF THE CAVE BEAR*

Jean Auel's (1980) insightful novel, *Clan of the Cave Bear*, clearly illustrates the mythical and archetypical qualities found in the cultural tales of wounded healers in prehistoric and ancient cultures, particularly the nurse as medicine woman. After witnessing the horrific death of her mother in an earthquake, three-year-old Ayla wanders away from her Cro-Magnon people through the frozen wastelands of Europe. Traumatized and overwhelmed with fear, she roams the countryside, surviving on local vegetation and suffering nightmares of her devastating loss.

During the journey, she inadvertently comes upon a pride of lions and is chased by one into a small dark cave. Extending a paw into the narrow cliff opening, the animal claws at her leg, leaving a large gaping wound that begins to fester. Severely injured physically as well as emotionally, Ayla remains in the hidden crevice throughout two days with her leg swollen, and enduring constant pain. Although delirious and dehydrated, she eventually manages to leave the hideaway and begins her quest for survival.

At that time, a group of Neanderthals, known as the Clan of the Cave Bear, are seeking a new site since their home has been destroyed by the quake. When Iza, the tribe's medicine woman observes Ayla lying on the ice, she convinces Brun the leader to allow her to rescue the child, who is dramatically different in appearance, being blond, blue-eyed, and comparatively verbal. Ayla is a marked contrast to her benefactors with their dark, coarse body hair, and the mixture of grunts and hand gestures they use to communicate.

Although she remains with the Clan members for several years, Ayla has never been completely accepted by them because of her unique appearance, advanced language skills, and mathematical ability. These aptitudes enrage Broud, the son of the group's leader, who molests and humiliates the young woman and turns the rest of the clan against her. Although the people empathize with Ayla's plight, no one intervenes to stop the violent abuse for fear of retribution.

Ayla survives by learning the ways of her adopted people, along with their use of herbs, incantations, and symbols. Iza and Creb—a revered, wounded shaman, crippled and partially blind from birth—become her patient mentors. Aware that she needs a strong totem to help her face life's difficulties, Creb designates the cave lion, one of the strongest spirits (never given to females), to be Ayla's protector even though the animal, ironically, has been the source of her initial wounding. Assigning a totem represents a common practice based on the assumption that a child may not reach maturity without the power of such a guardian spirit.

Although weapons are forbidden to women in the Neanderthal culture, Ayla breaks the rule by practicing secretly with a slingshot. One day when a hyena attacks a boy, she uses the implement to kill the beast. She then nurses the child back to health, administering medicine, cleaning the wound with an antiseptic solution, and setting his broken arm with dried birch bark.

By tribal law, these actions make her vulnerable to the death penalty, but because she has saved a life, the Clan condemns Ayla to the fate of a curse that usually results in the person's demise. After issuing this dictum, which banishes her from the cave for a period of one month, the people go about their chores and ignore her, a practice consistent with the curse. In their view, she now exists only among the spirits.

By using a small cave for shelter, Ayla endures the elements, becoming transformed and proving to herself that she can be self-sufficient. She returns to the community and eventually bears a son, Durc, who resembles a combination of the Clan and her Cro-Magnon heritage. At this point, realizing that the child is more like the Clan, she decides to leave the Neanderthals and find her own people. Only after departing and re-discovering her roots is she then able to transcend her earlier wounds of being different and isolated. As the forerunner of the nurse as wounded healer, Ayla accepts her own identity and becomes a great medicine woman.

HANA: *THE ENGLISH PATIENT*

Hana, the nurse protagonist in Michael Ondaatje's (1992) riveting work, *The English Patient*, clearly shows the development of the wounded healer. Having served in the armed forces during World War II, she recalls how an inner coldness, camouflaged by her role as a nurse, has helped sustain her when caring for seriously ill patients. "I will survive this, I won't fall apart," she tells herself (p. 48). Traumatized by the enormity of suffering that she describes as transporting "a ton of metal out of the huge body of human beings" (p. 50), Hana depersonalizes her interactions with the patients by calling each one "buddy" and viewing her exposure to them as "brief" and only "until death" (p. 51).

Nothing in her past experience has prepared her for such violence, especially witnessing a land mine explosion that kills another nurse. Filled with shame at what she has become and perceiving it as weakness, the young woman cannot face herself in the mirror.

When Hana begins to nurse the man referred to only as the English patient, she unknowingly begins the wounded healer's journey. Although immediately drawn to him, she does not consciously understand the attraction. During the hospital evacuation, she refuses to have the man transported far because of his severe burns. She decides to take him to an abandoned Italian villa, which she uses as a makeshift hospital to care for him. At first, her connection with the English patient appears somewhat distant because of the trauma incurred by the war, as well as her suffering from not being present when her father also died from severe burns.

Like Chiron the centaur, she uses the isolation of the villa to hide from her wounding, but it exists every day in the form of the English patient. Cutting her hair short and shedding her nurse's uniform appear to symbolize an incipient transformation. Yet, before it can occur, she must examine herself in this desolate setting.

Slightly confused by her situation, Hana reflects about her affinity for the patient, believing that something about him wants her "to learn, grow into, hide in, where she could turn away from being an adult" (p. 52). She is compelled to save this nameless, almost faceless man, one of the two hundred or so placed in her care during the invasion, and although recognizing the hopelessness of the situation, she meticulously attends to his every need. Through their relationship, she begins to express an unresolved grief and releases control. A dormant compassion emerges, and she submits to the English patient's desire to die by administering a lethal injection of morphine, an action that completely contradicts her nursing values.

Later, Hana realizes that in ministering to the English patient, she has been trying to attain power over a powerless situation, mindful of her father and his abandonment by the army unit that left him burned and wounded to die alone. Resurrecting this hurtful memory, she achieves an awareness of the root of her wounding declaring that "he was a burned man and I was a nurse and I could have nursed him. I could have saved him or at least been with him til the end" (p. 296). From such an epiphany, Hana attains a new level of growth through transcending her own pain. After the death of the English patient, which coincides with the end of the war, she becomes profoundly transformed and leaves the villa forever.

GEORGE BAILEY: *IT'S A WONDERFUL LIFE*

Set in the small American town of Bedford Falls, Frank Capra's 1946 allegorical film of a wounded healer chronicles the life of George Bailey. At the outset, Clarence Oddbody, Angel Second Class (ASC) learns that Bailey may be the last hope to earn his wings. Reviewing the man's history with his superior angel, Joseph, Clarence discovers that George, the oldest of two sons, was injured at the age of 12 after plunging into icy, cold waters to rescue his brother, Harry, and as a result developed deafness in the left ear.

The traumatic incident, however, does not deter him from living his life to the fullest. He first shows signs of being a healer when preventing Gower, the town druggist, from inadvertently poisoning a child due to a prescription error. Intoxicated after hearing the news that his young son died from influenza, Gower has carelessly put cyanide by mistake into the capsules. George's action results in saving the man from complete ruin and alcoholism.

Eager to achieve his long-time goals of going to college to study engineering and traveling abroad, Bailey's hopes are suddenly aborted just as he is about to leave for Europe. He discovers that Potter, the "richest and meanest man in town" intends to take over his deceased father's business, the Building and Loan Association, an outfit dedicated to helping working-class families purchase their own homes. As a consequence, he sacrifices the trip and postpones his studies to manage the company while giving the money for college to his younger brother. When Harry returns four years later as a married man, and unwilling to assume the reins of the family business, George's plans are again put on hold.

On the day that Bailey weds Mary, his childhood sweetheart, a financial crisis occurs when Potter tries to usurp control of the Building and Loan Association. Realizing that the community will be in jeopardy if such intentions materialize, George and Mary postpone their honeymoon and use their wedding money to quell the situation and save the business. Subsequently, a major crisis occurs when absent-minded Uncle Billy foolishly wraps an $8,000 deposit in a newspaper and hands it to Potter in a moment of distraction. Aware of the situation, the unscrupulous man steals the cash. When Uncle Billy realizes that the money is missing, he frantically searches for it, but in vain.

Learning about the loss, George panics because he understands the seriousness of the matter: it can cause the company's demise, a lengthy jail term, and the ruination of his entire family. Unable to locate the lost funds, rage and despair about his life of sacrifice consume him, and he verbally abuses Uncle Billy, his daughter's teacher, and his children. After drinking heavily, he crashes his car into a tree and contemplates suicide while standing on a bridge staring into the icy waters of the river, the source of his initial wounding in childhood.

Aware that he must intervene, Clarence appears and jumps into the water, crying out for assistance. George dives in to rescue him but continues to be cynical and scoffs at the explanation as to why their paths have crossed, especially because Clarence is not as yet a real angel. When the heavenly visitor recounts the details of Bailey's successful life, the despondent man responds, "I suppose it'd been better if I'd never been born at all."

This remark prompts the Angel Second Class to enlighten his companion about what the world would have been like without him. Their journey begins as the pair return to the site of the car crash, but no vehicle can be found. On entering the local bar, Bailey sees Gower, the druggist, now a hopeless drunk and ex-convict after poisoning a child with cyanide—all because George was not around to prevent the tragedy. George also observes that his hometown's name became Pottersville because he did not stop the hostile takeover.

Bedford Falls has turned into a decadent community with bars, burlesque houses, and gambling establishments lining the streets. George is stunned to discover his wife Mary as a spinster, his mother a bitter woman running a boarding house in town, and Uncle Billy, an institutionalized mental patient, committed after his failure to manage the family business. Even more startling is a gravestone inscribed with the date of his brother's death at the age of eight, since no one rescued the boy from the frozen lake.

Overwhelmed with what he has experienced, Bailey pleads with Clarence to let him live again, just as his friend Bert, the police officer, arrives to take him home. Mary and the children greet him, and within minutes their house becomes flooded with townspeople who bring all the money they can gather to help George raise the $8,000 and more. Their fine tribute to him makes him realize that he indeed has a wonderful life because of making it so for others, including Clarence, who finally acquires his wings.

This poignant story has particular relevance for nurses who often sacrifice themselves and do not acknowledge the vital contribution that they make to patients and society as a whole. When George stops to reflect on his own life, he achieves self-transcendence by acknowledging the good he had done for other human beings.

JIM: *LORD JIM*

Joseph Conrad's (1961) *Lord Jim* clearly explores many of the psychological issues involved in becoming a wounded healer, especially the difficulties with self-transcendence. The hero, a good-looking young man known only as Jim, lives in a vivid fantasy world that revolves around the search for fame and fortune. His dreams, however, cannot reach fruition because of his ambivalence about succeeding. He yearns to perform great deeds, but when an opportunity actually presents itself, he secretly is relieved when unable to achieve his high ideals.

Jim's vulnerability becomes apparent with his obsessive desire to go to sea. Fascinated by the relentless power of the ocean, he secures a position as assistant to the chief mate on a naval vessel. Toward the beginning of the voyage, a heavy part of the ship's mast falls on his head during a raging storm, but the effect of the injury, although moderately severe, is tempered by his inner joy at not having to engage in potentially dangerous deck activities during the tempest. Because of his slow recovery, Jim, like the mythical Philoctetes, remains on the island of Singapore to heal.

After recovering, the young man signs up to serve on the *Patna*, a rusty decaying ship, carrying 800 poor Moslem pilgrims traveling to holy sites in the Near East. Instead of heading for what should have been his Mecca, Jim's voyage on the steamer can be likened to a descent into the underworld, because he and the ship's unscrupulous crew abandon the *Patna* and its passengers when they believe it to be sinking. His shipmates disappear when reaching shore, leaving Jim alone to be prosecuted for desertion.

As a result of what is perceived as a cowardly action, he loses his British naval officer certification and any hope of commanding his own ship. However, as it turns out, the vessel had not sunk but was towed to safety with all the passengers unharmed. Reflecting on this traumatic episode, Jim's thoughts indicate his changed worldview as a trauma survivor, revealing that by abandoning his post he has "indeed jumped into an everlasting deep hole . . . tumbling from a height he could never scale again" (p. 87).

Finding it difficult to overcome his shame, he seeks solace in remote areas of the Far East, but is still haunted by the stigma of his actions which have become well known. Marlow, a sea captain twenty years his senior, befriends him, and introduces Jim to Mr. Stein, a wealthy trading post owner and entomologist with a particular interest in butterflies. After hearing Jim's story, Stein shares his own tale of facing death at one of his trading posts in a distant region. After escaping, Stein relates finding a rare butterfly and concludes that discovering the insect during the crisis symbolizes that something positive can emerge even when confronting life-threatening situations.

Eager to help Jim begin a new life and accept the foibles of his past, Stein suggests that he assume a post in Patusan, considered to be the most isolated place in the world. At one time, the area was a lucrative site for pepper, but eventually its popularity decreased because of other more accessible regions for harvesting the spice.

Jim's endeavor achieves a marked success making him so beloved by the Bugi natives that they refer to him as Lord Jim. When Marlow later visits him at the outpost, he observes at once the change in Jim, who has developed more self-acceptance by helping the people to grow and become more productive. Although confronted by warring factions in the land led by Sherif Ali, a guerrilla terrorist, Jim is determined to promote peace and decides to hoist two huge brass canons up a huge mountain to destroy Ali's camp on an opposite hill. After accomplishing this great feat, he is more revered than ever and viewed as a godlike figure. By reclaiming responsibility for others, the wounding incurred from the earlier *Patna* incident seems to have diminished.

Toward the end of Jim's quest, he has been transformed by his own experience into a man of true honor and integrity. When an opportunity arises to destroy Gentleman Brown and the other pirates who intrude upon the land, he refuses although the invaders have been greatly outnumbered by the natives. Lord Jim allows Brown to leave peacefully, making the promise that if any harm came to the Bugi, he will sacrifice his own life. Brown's unscrupulousness, however, betrays this trust when he launches a surprise attack on one of the villages, killing many inhabitants. With his fate sealed, Jim is murdered by one of the native chieftains.

The characterization of the hero in *Lord Jim* becomes defined when he succeeds in transforming himself into the wounded healer by rising above his failings. Roberts (1986) elaborates on the growth of Jim and his evolution as follows:

> Being a Lord to his people, he had to give his life when it was necessary. This time he did not flee, he did not jump. He had conquered the

fear and shame and met death as a hero would. He made a bargain with the human community, a community he once deserted, and he paid for its trust with his own life. At last, Jim became a master of his own destiny (pp. 77–78).

CELIE: *THE COLOR PURPLE*

Celie, the major character in Alice Walker's (1982) *The Color Purple* reflects the author's personal odyssey as she travels the path to successful transcendence. Partially blind from childhood as a result of a BB gun accident, Walker also had to endure extreme poverty and racism. Barbara Christian (1998), a professor of African-American studies at the University of California, frames the novel as a slave narrative that parallels the wounded healer archetype, showing the heroine's growing awareness of the trauma inherent in oppression, her increasing resistance and escape, and her final realization of freedom in body and spirit.

A plain black woman living in the early twentieth century, Celie, the main character, comes from a family in which her father has been lynched and her mother becomes mentally ill after remarrying an insensitive, violent man. On his wife's death, Celie's stepfather takes over the family home with no intention of sharing it with the rightful heirs. Celie is repeatedly exposed to the abuse of her stepfather and bears his two children, who are forcibly removed and given away to unknown adoptive parents. The emotional suffering that follows creates a state of isolation which limits her ability to relate openly.

Celie's stepfather sells her to "Mister," a black man, whom she cares for along with his two children. He becomes abusive and tries to seduce her younger sister, Nettie, who eventually runs away. From Nettie, she has learned to read and write which helps her to remain connected to the outside world. She writes to her sister every day, and when the letters go unanswered, she assumes that Nettie is dead.

In time, Celie meets Shug Avery, Mister's blues-singing friend from Memphis, and they form a close bond. Through this loving relationship, she begins to accept herself, marking the beginning of her transformation. Shug discovers that Nettie had written to Celie for many years as promised but that Mister had hidden the letters. When uncovering them, they learn that Nettie has located her sister's children on a trip to Africa where they live with adoptive missionary parents.

Celie's search leads to Memphis to live with Shug where she acquires economic independence by initiating her own clothing business. Through this transition, she develops the insight to transcend the years of pain and heals herself and the community. Eventually even Mister undergoes some transformation and approaches her to help him make clothing. A poignant event takes place at a Fourth of July picnic when Celie is reunited with her children and sister and gains possession of her father's house.

The title, The Color Purple, connotes some symbolism in that the hue appears much more commonly in nature than realized. To some degree, its beauty can always be recognized although blended into the background.

RANDALL PATRICK MCMURPHY: ONE FLEW OVER THE CUCKOO'S NEST

A facinating picture of irony emerges in Ken Kesey's novel in which the patients evolve into wounded healers, while the head nurse, Mildred Ratched, conversely becomes the antihealer by virtue of her cruel and inhumane treatment of the patients. As the Big Nurse, she represents the Shadow on a long-term psychiatric hospital ward where her "healing" relationships with patients are characterized by domination, control, and rigidity. Impeccably garbed in her white starched uniform, she administers medications and performs group therapy as she deems fit, displaying her unyielding power trip.

The central character, Randall Patrick McMurphy, labeled a psychopath, has been committed to the institution after experiencing some "hassles at the work farm" (Kesey, 1996, p. 13). Most of the other patients have voluntarily admitted themselves into the milieu, reinforcing a dependency counterproductive to achieving a healthy status. As such, they accept Nurse Ratched's preference for prescriptive healing at the expense of developing self-responsibility. Although Ratched shows extreme anger when functioning on the ward, the woman cleverly portrays herself as a caring, helpful nurse, especially in the presence of the psychiatrists who defer to her judgment on clinical and various other matters.

From the outset of McMurphy's admission, all the inmates, especially Chief Bromden, view him differently from the others. Bromden, a strapping Native American patient who is a war veteran and victim of racial discrimination comes to the ward in a psychotic and nonverbal state. To escape his shattered life, he remains mute while perceiving the life around him through a cloud. Eventually, McMurphy heals the man as well as an autistic patient through his straightforwardness and by using himself as a therapeutic instrument.

Because McMurphy does not participate in the "sick games" that pass for therapy on the ward, a power struggle ensues between him and the head nurse. When a crisis triggered by Ratched results in the suicide of a young patient, he loses his temper and brutally assaults her. Although bruised and battered as a result of the attack, she appears relatively unaffected on her return to work the following day. In reality, it is she and not McMurphy that represents the quintessential psychopath with seemingly no awareness or remorse as to how her own behavior contributed to the boy's death.

McMurphy's capacity to reach some of the patients helps them recover and leave the institution. Although the opportunity arises at one point for him to escape, he determines his own fate by refusing to abandon the remaining patients. When electric shock treatments are ordered because of his defiant behavior, he resists them successfully but his insubordination is eventually quelled permanently by undergoing a lobotomy.

By the end of the drama an interesting twist emerges because his sacrifice, like Chiron with Prometheus, allows the healing of others to take place. Through McMurphy's efforts, Chief Bromden has transcended his trauma and becomes the wounded healer. When he sees the man that he has admired so much in a lobotomized and vegetative state, he finds the sight unbearable and suffocates him. A transformed Bromden then literally breaks through the barred institutional windows confining him and disappears into the sunset.

MARGARET HOULIHAN: *MOBILE ARMY SURGICAL HOSPITAL: M*A*S*H*

The transformation of Major Margaret Houlihan RN, chief nurse of the 4077th M*A*S*H,* occurs over a period of time with noticeable milestones. Born into a military lifestyle, she has moved frequently during her childhood, finding it difficult to cope with the loss of friends and acquaintances. Her decision to follow the family tradition of the armed service may be admirable, but it has also been restrictive.

Rarely can she exhibit vulnerability to others because it has been so strongly discouraged in her early upbringing, as exemplified by her father's wedding gift of a gun to his new bride! Margaret follows the Houlihan tradition of being serious about officers' training and nursing school. When she goes to war-ravaged Korea to practice nursing and to advance her army career, the action represents the beginning of her search for self.

The nickname "Hot Lips" indicates the original perception of her as a sex symbol rather than a competent nurse. Indoctrinated with the notion of "clean hands perfection," her approach to caring usually stems from following rules and regulations rather than human feelings and empathetic connections. This character trait emerges frequently in her relationships with colleagues, manifested by temper tantrums if assignments or procedures are not followed according to the book—and with ultimate solemnity.

Margaret's lack of self-worth becomes apparent in her continuing affair with Frank Burns, a married man, which makes her the target of ridicule among most of the male officers. In retaliation, she reports them to the commanding officer for any slight infraction of the rules. An angry woman, she cannot face herself and lashes out at the other nurses as they, in turn, remain detached from her. At one point, her pain shows through while chastising them for excluding her from their inner circle.

Margaret cannot concede that it is her own woundedness and inability to form healthy relationships that perpetuates the problem. These feelings are revealed in the bitterness of her question to the nurses: "*Did you ever once show me friendship? Ever ask my help in a personal problem? Include me in one of your little bull sessions?*" she asks. "*Can you imagine how it feels to walk by this tent and hear your laughter and know that I'm not welcome? When did one of you ever offer me a lousy cup of coffee?*" (Kalter, 1984, p. 107). When the nurses reply that they didn't think Margaret would accept, she simply states that they are wrong and does not pursue the matter further, while retaining her resentment.

Most of the time she succeeds in concealing her true caring nature, which appears to surface only when away from other colleagues. In one M*A*S*H* episode, Margaret fearlessly leaves the safety of the camp and faces capture by enemy forces to deliver a Korean villager's baby. In another instance, she breaks a cardinal rule of procedure by helping the surgeons to falsify the date of the death certificate of a soldier so that his family will not always associate the event with Christmas Day. However, when performing patient-focused tasks, she always demonstrates marked empathy.

A turning point in Margaret's life occurs when she is granted a requested transfer because of her disappointment and bitterness regarding the lack of fulfillment in both her personal and professional life. During her farewell celebration, she becomes intoxicated just as the helicopters bring in more wounded who need her in the OR. Hawkeye, one of the surgeons, wryly informs her that he has ordered a new type of surgical prep, namely, "a scrub from head to toe with her clothes on" to help sober her up! (Kalter, 1984, p. 58) She begins to understand that her colleagues care for her and expresses her appreciation, exhibiting a marked change in attitude.

Finally, realizing that Frank Burns will never leave his wife for her, Margaret ends the relationship and becomes engaged to another army officer. Before the wedding, however, symptoms of trauma surface in one of her dreams where her wedding gown drips with blood and the marriage bed becomes an operating table. Feelings of helplessness arise on spotting an empty tray as she attempts to give the surgeon an instrument. When the marriage later ends, she acknowledges that the time has arrived to take stock of her life and help herself to heal the emotional wounding that has been intensified in the ongoing war.

During one incident, the entire unit seeks shelter in a cave because of enemy fire but after some consideration, Margaret and Hawkeye return to the camp to save a boy's life. By assuming full responsibility as the chief nurse, she indicates an ability to transcend her fear by stating, "I'll be damned if I'm going to send someone else out to face what terrifies me!" (Kalter, 1984, p. 149).

Before leaving Korea, she reveals more of her humanity and no longer allows herself to be the target of sexual innuendo. Instead, she socializes with the rest of the group, laughs at herself, and even mends her long-time feud with Hawkeye. While preparing to return to the States with the war ending, she is flattered when Winchester, another surgeon, gives her a book of sonnets by Elizabeth Barrett Browning, one of his prized possessions. Through her experiences at the 4077th, Margaret Houlihan has acquired an awareness of her true nature and emerges transformed as a respected professional, more secure with herself and admired by colleagues.

JOHN COFFEY: *THE GREEN MILE*

Stephen King's (1996) esoteric tale concerning a wounded healer and new inmate John Coffey is narrated from the perspective of Paul Edgecombe, the supervisor of death row located in Cell Block E at the Cold Mountain Penal Institution. Most prison employees refer to the death row unit as the "Green Mile" rather than the Last Mile because the wide central corridor is "floored with linoleum the color of tired old limes" (p. 6). Edgecombe focuses on Coffey, whom he finds to be unusual, and notes that "once his eyes found me, they never left me" (p. 12).

A slow-witted black man of great height measuring six feet, eight inches tall and weighing over 300 pounds, Coffey has been sentenced to death for the murder of nine-year-old twin girls. Incarcerated after being discovered on a river bank with the limp bodies of the children in his arms, he repeatedly cries out that he "couldn't help it" and he "tried to take it back but couldn't" (p. 349). At first, his words are interpreted as a confession, but later Edgecombe discovers that Coffey found their corpses and tried unsuccessfully to heal them (p. 350). Although little is known about Coffey's background, it appears that he has been abused, as revealed by the deep scars on his arms and back.

Unknown to his captors at first, the prisoner shows unusual skills after spotting Edgecombe in pain from a severe urinary tract infection that has not responded to treatment. Observing his agony, Coffey summons Edgecombe to his cell and then pins him against the cell bars while grabbing and holding the supervisor's groin for a short period of time. This action cures the infection instantly, and when the prisoner coughs, he expels a black cloud of swarming flies that turn white and disappear into a harmless white dust. The treatment appears to symbolize that Coffey has drawn the illness into himself, and then released and transformed it.

Amazed by the seeming paradox of healer and killer, Edgecombe decides to investigate the man's crime. After consulting with the defense attorney on the case, he becomes more certain that Coffey is not guilty upon observing him resurrect another inmate's pet mouse crushed to near death by the evil guard Percy.

When Edgecombe shares his own healing experience with three other guards in the cell block, they are astonished by the "miracle" and help him smuggle Coffey out of the prison under cover of darkness to cure the warden's wife who is afflicted with a brain tumor. On meeting the prisoner, she inquires about the numerous scars on his hands and arms, and asks who hurt him so badly. He can only reply that he didn't "rightly remember where they all came from" (p. 406).

Like a shaman removing the impurities out of a sick individual, Coffey extracts the negative elements of her disease into himself, but does not expel anything at the time. After being completely healed, she embraces him and he returns to the prison. He then releases the swarm into the mouth of the evil guard, who in turn shoots and kills Wharton, a violent inmate.

When asked why he has committed this act, Coffey grabs Edgecombe's arm and conveys to him a vision of how the two little girls had been murdered by Wharton. Convinced of the man's innocence, Edgecombe realizes that no one else will believe the fantastic story. He is willing to risk his job to release Coffey, but the prisoner refuses because he is weary of the world's enduring pain and instead chooses to submit to the death sentence.

While Coffey is being strapped to the electric chair, the other guards who have been transformed by the happenings, vow never again to be part of the violence of execution and resign their jobs. Edgecombe also leaves the prison to work with troubled youth and intervene before criminality becomes ingrained. As the wounded healer, John Coffey sacrifices himself so that others will know the true meaning of life.

JUDAH BEN-HUR: *BEN HUR: A TALE OF THE CHRIST*

In his classic work published in 1880, Lew Wallace epitomizes the wounded healer in the main character Judah Ben-Hur, a wealthy Jewish prince living in Jerusalem during Christ's public ministry. Judah enjoys a charmed and prosperous life until he reconnects with his boyhood friend, Messala, a Roman who is determined to crush Jewish resistance in Palestine. Messala urges him to betray his countrymen by providing the names of Jewish conspirators to the Roman authorities. He becomes angry when Ben-Hur refuses, and attempts to eliminate him by false accusations about attempting to murder a prominent official.

Messala's evil knows no bounds as he condemns Judah's entire family to cruel punishment in order to make examples of them to the rest of the rebels. After being imprisoned for a short time, Ben-Hur escapes and intends to kill Messala, but when threatened with the crucifixion of his mother and sister, he chooses to sacrifice himself for their lives. Although sentenced to become a galley slave, a fate offering no return for the condemned, he remains resolute to stay alive and seek revenge on Messala.

On the way to the ship where he will be imprisoned, the caravan stops at Nazareth. The guards refuse to give Judah anything to drink, but on meeting Jesus who offers him water, his captors are reluctant to forbid it. Ben-Hur then becomes convinced of his survival, symbolizing a beginning transformation.

The galley in the Roman battleship represents the underworld or descent into hell where the chained men must endure the whip with little possibility of escape. When the Roman officer Quintus Arrius notices Judah's defiance, he admires it and instructs the guard to remove his chains during a naval battle. Grateful to the younger man for rescuing him when he falls overboard, he adopts Ben-Hur and brings him to Rome to become a citizen. Dissatisfied after awhile with his new identity, "Young Arrius" returns to Palestine to find himself and seek revenge on his enemy.

Following the great chariot race, the moribund Messala informs Judah of his mother's and sister's imprisonment in a dungeon, where they have developed leprosy. Shattered by this revelation, he goes to the Valley of the Lepers and touches his family regardless of the potential harm to himself. Encouraged by Esther, the daughter of one of his former employees, Ben-Hur agrees to bring them to see Jesus with the hope of being healed, but on the way they learn that the man is about to be crucified.

Judah recognizes Christ as the person that gave him water in the desert four years earlier. While witnessing the crucifixion, his healing reaches fruition as he states, "Almost at the moment he died, I heard Him say 'Father, forgive them for they know not what they do' and I felt His voice take the sword out of my hand" (Zimbalist & Wyler, 1959). Following this spiritual awakening and with renewed faith, he discovers that his mother and sister have been healed of their disease and the family becomes whole again. Conscious of a change in his feelings, Judah Ben-Hur acquires a conception of "something better than the best of his life—something so much better that it could serve a weak man with strength to endure the agonies of the spirit as well as of the body" (Wallace, 1978, p. 830).

REFERENCES

Auel, J. M. (1980). *The clan of the cave bear.* New York: Bantam Books.

Capra, F. (Producer & Director). (1946). *It's a wonderful life* [Videocassette]. Available from Goodtimes Homevideo, 401 Fifth Avenue, New York, NY, 10016.

Christian, B. (1998). *Monarch notes: Alice Walker's The Color Purple.* New York: Simon & Schuster.

Conrad, J. (1961). *Lord Jim.* New York: Doubleday. (Original work published 1899)

Kalter, S. (1984). *The complete book of* M.A.S.H. New York: Abrams.

Kesey, K. (1996). *One flew over the cuckoo's nest.* New York: Penguin. (Original work published in 1962).

King, S. (1996). *The green mile: The complete serial novel.* New York: Pocket Books.

Ondaatje, M. (1992). *The English patient.* New York: Vintage.

Roberts, J. L. (1986). *Cliff's notes on Conrad's Lord Jim.* Lincoln, NE: Cliff's Notes.

Walker, A. (1982). *The color purple.* New York: Harcourt, Brace Jovanovich.

Wallace, L. (1978). *Ben-Hur: A tale of the Christ.* New York: Bonanza. (Original work published 1880)

Zimbalist, S. (Producer) & Wyler, W. (Director). (1959). *Ben-Hur* [Videocassette]. Available from MGM/UA Home Video, Inc., 1000 Washington Boulevard, Culver City, CA 90232.

CHAPTER 8

FACTUAL PORTRAYALS OF THE WOUNDED HEALER

HARRIET ROSS TUBMAN (1820–1913)

Primarily known for her heroic role in founding the Underground Railroad during the Civil War, Harriet Ross Tubman, the "Moses of her people," was not only a nurse but a spy for the Union Army (Bradford, 1993). Traveling on many perilous trips, she succeeded in rescuing over 300 slaves including her parents and a number of siblings.

A descendant of the Ashanti people of West Africa, Harriet was born into slavery in Bucktown, Maryland, often enduring severe beatings throughout her childhood (Bullough, Church, & Stein, 1988). Forced to work as a plantation laborer beginning at the age of five, she had no formal education, few clothes to wear, and little to eat. In response to these unfortunate circumstances, she became defiant and rebellious.

As a teenager, she suffered a fractured skull from a lead weight thrown by a cruel overseer who was attempting to stop her from helping a runaway (Sahlman, 2000). The injury resulted in a coma and lengthy recovery, along with serious consequences producing pain and spells of narcolepsy. The episodes often occurred under the most dangerous of conditions even when Harriet was transporting slaves to freedom (Brewer, 1978).

At 24, she married a freed black man, John Tubman, but still had to retain her slave status. Fearful of being sent further south to be sold, the young woman escaped north to Philadelphia, leaving her husband behind (Sahlman, 2000). This dangerous journey transformed her life, laying the preparation for the Underground Railroad.

Described as barely five feet tall, Harriet had the thick strong muscles of a field hand, a prominent scar on her temple, and a husky voice from an earlier bout with bronchitis (Brewer, 1978, p. 3). Resolute in her purpose, she warned the escapees about the risks involved, which meant that they would "have to go through the ordie" (Harriet Tubman Home, 2000). Using the North Star as a guide, they traveled by night, climbing surreptitiously over mountains, crossing dangerous rivers, and hiding from the bounty hunters. Babies, carried in baskets on Tubman's arms, were drugged with paregoric to prevent them from crying (Bradford, 1993).

So stressful was the journey that the exhausted men would fall to the ground, yearning to give up and return to their homes. Bolstered by her deep faith in God's assistance, Harriet threatened to kill any of the runaways if they gave in to cowardice and attempted to turn back. Fully aware that a living person could reveal secrets, she once pointed a gun at one of her charges and threatened, "Dead folks tell no tales" (Sterling & Logan, 1967, p. 16). She elaborated as follows:

> There were one or two things I had the right to, liberty or death. If I could not have one, I would have the other, for no man should take me alive. I should fight for my liberty as long as my strength lasted, and when the time came for me to go, the Lord would let them take me. (Bradford, 1993, p. 29)

During the Civil War, blacks rescued by the Union Army to escape Southern oppression were regarded as contraband. Accorded this status, Tubman was recruited into military service as a hospital nurse, working under primitive conditions while caring for both white and black patients as she moved from camp to camp. Although exposed to dysentery, malaria, smallpox, and malignant fevers, she never became ill, having been endowed with both the physical and spiritual strength to sustain her (Fowler, 1978).

With dysentery prevalent and the cause of many deaths, the resourceful Harriet used her knowledge of roots and herbs to seek a cure. When stationed in South Carolina, she took a boat inland and searched until she found some water lilies, plants commonly found in her native Maryland (Brewer, 1978). By brewing the roots into a bitter tasting tea, she made an effective remedy to treat the illness. Her ability to prepare other herbal medicines also led to saving numerous lives.

Much of Tubman's later years after the war were spent in poverty until the federal government awarded her a pension. She moved to Auburn, New York, using her own home as a shelter for needy and sick black people. In 1897, Queen Victoria honored her with the silver medal for bravery, one of the many accolades she eventually received (Sahlman, 2000).

Harriet Tubman's inspiring story represents one of trauma and transformation, as well as slave to freewoman, as graphically described in her own words: "I looked in my hands to see if I was the same person now that I was free. There was such a glory over everything; The sun came like gold through the trees and over the fields and I felt like I was in heaven" (Bradford, 1993, p. 30).

FLORENCE NIGHTINGALE (1820–1910)

With the enduring fame ascribed to Florence Nightingale, how many people would think of this strong-minded and accomplished woman as typifying the wounded healer archetype? Yet, an examination of various happenings occurring over time reveal some marked credibility to this notion. Named after the city of her birth in Italy, she spent her early years at Lea Hurst, living in the family manor near Derbyshire in Northern England (Siegel, 1991). This period of her life, however, was not a happy one for Florence, who felt "lonely and different," and gave vent to moods of intense anger and sullenness (Siegel, 1991, p. 16).

Preoccupied with extensive daydreaming, she fantasized becoming a heroine like Joan of Arc (Siegel, 1991). Although Florence came from an aristocratic background, she rejected many of the social obligations of the rich, and preferred to follow her own inclinations. Her initial exposure to nursing occurred when she accompanied her mother to a neighboring village where they brought food, clothing, and medicine to the poor and needy.

While still a young girl, Florence expressed a desire to become a nurse, but such aspirations seemed remote in light of her family's status in English society. Nevertheless, a spiritual awakening occurred when she was sixteen which reinforced her hopes. She reported, "God spoke to me and called me to his service" (Siegel, 1991, p. 22). Following this experience, she began to tend the local indigent population for a few months in the belief that her behavior stemmed from God wanting her to perform nursing work. It was of some consequence when Florence admitted that being one with Christ and following his will gave her a sense of woundedness in carrying out her mission in life (Montgomery-Dossey, 2000).

Family opposition to her interest in preparing for nursing formed the basis of the trauma that plagued Nightingale for a long time. Initially, she had been more deeply affected by the oppression of wealth than poverty because of the restrictions it created on her life (Siegel, 1991). Independent and determined, she left for Kaiserworth in her mid-twenties to study with the deaconnesses in caring for the sick, released prisoners, and orphans. Unable, however, to carry out her plans to continue nursing when she returned to England, she became seriously depressed. Concerned, the family sent her to recover on the continent in Greece and Italy, which proved to be the therapeutic sojourn needed prior to embarking on her journey to the Crimea.

It was wartime and Scutari became Nightingales's quest into the "underworld," with the appalling conditions of the Barrack Hospital and the injuries, rampant disease, and deaths of the patients. Rather than give in to despair, she used her own money as well as funds collected from other sources to obtain the necessary supplies and equipment. Working indefatigably around the clock, she coordinated and participated in the renovation of the hospital, while enforcing strict guidelines for nursing care and conduct.

Weary from spending long hours administering the facility's operation and working with great intensity caring for the soldiers, Nightingale's health began to suffer. During the war, she endured many illnesses, including dysentery and Crimean fever (brucellosis), which produced attacks of weakness, palpitations, dizziness, and joint pain (Montgomery-Dossey, 1998). Other conditions such as neurasthenia, chronic fatigue, or rheumatoid arthritis could also not be discounted. Furthermore, a strong possibility existed that Nightingale suffered posttraumatic stress disorder after experiencing the horrific conditions at Scutari because she seemed haunted afterward by memories of the ordeal (Harbart & Hunsinger, 1991).

At the age of thirty-seven, she became physically incapacitated and declared herself an invalid, putting limits on her time and health that were interfering with her sole mission in life devoted to reform work (Montgomery-Dossey, 2000). After retreating for a while to the ancestral home at Embley Park, she rented a suite of rooms at the Burlington Hotel Annex in London and in 1865 moved to a house on South Street, which became her permanent residence. In a sense, typical of the wounded healer, she chose to spend most of her time in a symbolic cave to achieve her goals.

During the post-Crimean years (1856–1861), she was able to effect lasting social change through her greatest accomplishments, including the establishment of the nursing school at St. Thomas Hospital and the Royal Commission for the reform of the army, as well as the development of public health standards in England and India (Selanders, 1998, p. 233). Around this period, she published *Notes on Nursing* and *Notes on Hospitals*, both considered seminal works.

In the early 1860s, Nightingale's wounding reemerged to some extent when she encountered roadblocks to her health care reform because of the male-dominated Victorian society in which she lived. Her effectiveness was also curtailed by the deaths of her allies, Sir Sidney Herbert and Lord Palmerston. Nevertheless, she ultimately achieved self-transcendence in later years, recognizing her contributions and taking more of an interest in her family (Montgomery-Dossey, 2000).

Florence Nightingale's journey has been likened to a mystic's quest, culminating in transformation and transcendence (Montgomery-Dossey, 2000). How well she achieved her mission is best revealed in her own statement:

> Thirty nine years ago [I] arrived at Scutari. The immense blessings I have had . . . the longings of my heart accomplished . . . and now drawn to Thee by difficulties and disappointments. Homeward bound I have entered in. (Cook, 1913, p. 415)

CARL GUSTAV JUNG (1875–1961)

Carl Gustav Jung, the renowned psychiatrist, can be credited as the major figure responsible for bringing the wounded healer archetype into modern consciousness. Born into a well-educated Swiss family in 1875, he lived modestly in an eighteenth-century parsonage where his father was a country clergyman (Dunne, 2000).

Young Carl had his first serious traumatic experience at the age of three when turmoil in his parent's marriage erupted, resulting in his mother's being hospitalized in a mental institution. Deeply troubled by her absence, he suffered bouts of eczema after being sent away temporarily to live with an aunt

(Dunne, 2000; McLynn, 1996). Following his mother's release, her frequent bouts of depression, dissociation, and mood swings disturbed him markedly, and set up a pattern of distrusting women that never left him (Jung, 1989).

Traumatic incidents continued to plague Jung throughout his lifetime. He became "accident-prone," sustaining a number of injuries, such as falling down a flight of stairs and later burning himself so badly on a stove that the wound remained visible until young adulthood (McLynn, 1996). This pattern probably stemmed from a fear of death and extreme anxiety that may have been engendered by the morbid prayers that his mother recited to him every evening. She would allude to Jesus "eating" his "little chicks" (children) so that Satan would not devour them! (McLynn, 1996, p. 10).

Jung (1989) began to rebel against the Lord Jesus of his childhood prayers, transferring his suspicions onto the local Jesuit priests who came to symbolize Christ. He eventually rejected organized religion and opted to study symbols, myths, and spirituality, influences that would greatly affect the development of his psychological theories.

As a boy, the tendency toward his emotional wounding intensified when at the age of eleven, he attended a school far from home where he felt "different and alienated" (Dunne, 2000, p. 10). This sense of isolation became magnified by an awareness of his relative poverty as compared to the material wealth of his schoolmates. Yet, the fact that Jung had acquired some distance from his parents, enabled him to achieve a certain level of insight into his traumatic family life. He could recall being emotionally torn between them and forced to mediate their arguments. His mother had also aggravated this parentification pattern by confiding in him rather than her husband (Jung, 1989).

When he turned twelve, Carl began to have "neurotic fainting spells" after "striking his head against a curbstone following an attack by fellow student" (Jung, 1989, p. 30). He learned to use the symptoms to his advantage, however, by avoiding certain activities in school like gym and by gaining sympathy from his family. After a physician suggested that epilepsy might be the cause of the disturbing behavior, Jung feared that he would be marred for life and unable to work as a result of the diagnosis. To overcome the spells, he sat in a chair and repeatedly told himself that he would not faint. As a consequence, he understood the repercussions of neurosis and never succumbed to the episodes again (Jung, 1989).

The traumatic circumstances of his earlier years motivated him to study medicine and focus his doctoral thesis on psychology, pathology, and occult phenomena. Selecting what was viewed as controversial topics drew criticism from his teacher and colleagues, once again added to his wounding. Nevertheless, he began to achieve more understanding of himself and could proceed on the desired path.

Jung's approach to treating patients seemed unique for the times because instead of focusing on diagnoses, symptoms, and statistics, he listened to the individual's personal stories and dreams and integrated them into the context in which they took place (Dunne, 2000). His methods, including a word association technique, eventually brought him great recognition in the treatment of schizophrenia.

Although Jung married at the age of 28, his most significant relationship occurred with Sigmund Freud, who regarded him as a son and heir (Dunne, 2000). Their association flourished over a period of seven years, conducted mainly through correspondence. Because of their closeness, Jung was able to confess to his mentor that he had been sexually abused by a man at the age of eighteen (McLynn, 1996).

In time, the relationship with Freud dissipated when they began to espouse opposing views. Jung's belief that the causes of certain pathological tendencies were unrelated to sexuality but rather related to factors such as environment, challenged the theories expounded by Freud, and conflict ensued between them (Jung, 1989). By 1913, they ceased speaking with one another after Jung's views on incest and mysticism became the central focus of disagreement (Dunne, 2000, pp. 43–44).

The choice to become his own person may have appeared sound, but it left him deeply troubled and led to a serious breakdown. During this period, he fantasized floods sweeping over Europe, which seemed to foreshadow the coming of war (Dunne, 2000). He also experienced visions, dreams, and inner voices, including one alluding to a dark cave (Dunne, 2000).

Remembering when he cured himself of the fainting spells as a boy, Jung consciously started to work on his own self-transcendence. As a daily practice, he analyzed his inner thoughts by drawing circles containing certain images. Known as *mandalas*, the Sanskrit word for "circle," they symbolized, "the state of the self that presented anew to him each day" (Jung, 1989, p. 196). Through this process, he came to understand that the goal of psychic development was the self, an insight that gave him stability and inner peace (Jung, 1989). As a result of his experiences, he concluded that "only the wounded physician heals" and then "only to the extent that he has healed himself" (Jung, 1989, p. 134).

Transformed from the journey within, he extended his search to traveling to other lands to study native peoples. From these explorations, he more clearly delineated the field of Analytical Psychology, a system broad in scope. He deduced that through intensive examination of the structural as well as functional components of the personality, the individual can integrate both the conscious and the unconscious mind. Jung perceived transcendence as recognizing and rising above the opposing forces in human nature and the ability to see all aspects of the person (Boeree, 1997).

Before his death, Carl Jung, the "wounded healer of the soul" (Dunne, 2000), offered these illuminating comments: "We have learned to place in the foreground of the personality of the practitioner himself, as a curative or harmful factor; what is now demanded is his own transformation—the self-education of the educator" (Jung, 1929, p. 74).

ANNA ELEANOR ROOSEVELT (1884–1962)

The woundedness of Anna Eleanor Roosevelt had its roots early in her life. Although she came from a prominent New York family that claimed Theodore Roosevelt as a close relative, she was exposed to the trauma of an alcoholic father and the cruelty of maternal emotional abuse: her mother referred to her as "granny" to denote her plain appearance. Although named after her handsome mother, she was always called Nell or Eleanor, and never forgot the suggestion that she needed to create manners to make up for her poor looks (Wiesen-Cook, 1992).

As a child, Eleanor patterned her life in response to the problems of her parents believing that if she did well, it would make them happy and prevent emotional abandonment (Wiesen-Cook, 1992). The rejection encountered during this formative period made her painfully shy, a trait she vowed to overcome. It also left her with a deep sense of insecurity and inadequacy and the need for praise and affection. In time, however, she developed the capacity to empathize with people in need from all walks of life.

When Eleanor was eight years old, her twenty-nine-year-old mother passed away from complications of diphtheria, and two years later, her father died as a result of his alcoholism. Since Eleanor loved her father dearly, this loss caused a deep wound. After living with her maternal grandmother until the age of fifteen, she was sent to an elite European boarding school. On returning to New York, her desire to help the more unfortunate began to evolve, and she became interested in social work on the Lower East Side. The crowded environment of the garment district exposed her to the shocking conditions of the laboring class, where she witnessed small children forced to work long hours until they collapsed from exhaustion. During World War I, she also visited wounded soldiers, an experience that moved her greatly and helped shape her future altruistic activities.

The hurtful experiences of her childhood continued when she married her distant cousin Franklin Delano Roosevelt (FDR). His mother, Sara, dominated the union by attempting to control all aspects of the household including the raising of the six grandchildren. Eleanor also endured the painful loss of a seventh infant child from influenza. At the same time, Franklin spent so much time preparing for his political career that she often felt abandoned. When she unwittingly came across some amorous correspondence between FDR and Lucy Mercer, her social secretary, the revelations devastated her. Nevertheless, in spite of the affair, the couple agreed to remain married. From that point on, however, Eleanor began to transform her feelings of betrayal by concentrating on her own life and goals, working independently with such organizations as the League of Women Voters and the Women's Union League (Micrsoft® Encarta® Online Encyclopedia, 2000).

When FDR was stricken with poliomyelitis at the age of thirty-nine, it created a crisis in his career, but an opportunity arrived for Eleanor to become more influential in his political life. After he became President in 1932 during the Great Depression, she devoted her time to the broader social issues such as the unemployment of West Virginia coal miners and the problems of the youth of the nation.

One of Mrs. Roosevelt's more ennobling acts, which provided strong role modeling in the area of racial discrimination, included her resignation from the Daughters of the American Revolution (DAR) when the group denied

Marian Anderson, a prominent black singer, the right to sing in one of their establishments. She wrote to the DAR protesting their attitude in refusing the artist's appearance in Constitution Hall: "You had an opportunity to lead in an enlightened way and it seems to me that your organization has failed," she noted (A&E Television Network, 2000). As a result of this action, the federal government invited Anderson to sing in front of the Lincoln Memorial on Easter Sunday in 1939 before a crowd of over 75,000 people. Her performance of "My Country 'Tis of Thee" turned out to be one of the most inspiring events in the nation's history, (A&E Television Network, 1994).

During the thirties, Eleanor Roosevelt's personal healing was facilitated in part by a number of friends including Lorena Hickock, a well known-reporter who helped her transform the trauma of early rejection. Hickock assisted in instituting weekly press conferences attended only by female journalists, and encouraged her to write a daily newspaper column entitled *My Day*, which focused on the First Lady's view of important political and social issues. The series became syndicated in over 180 publications nationwide.

As World War II approached, Eleanor became even more active as Franklin's political partner, traveling abroad to give support and encouragement to the troops. An advocate of desegregation in the military, she also championed the placement of European Jewish refugees in Palestine when the war ended.

In addition to her grief when the President died, Eleanor suffered deep wounding after learning that his relationship had been rekindled with Lucy Mercer, who was with Roosevelt at the time of his death. With typical dignity, she stood by the side of his successor, Harry Truman during the swearing in ceremony.

An impressive part of Eleanor Roosevelt's legacy lies in her contribution to the United Nations Universal Declaration of Human Rights, which was adopted during her appointment as U.N. Ambassador from the United States. The document reflects her ongoing struggle for the rights of others, which emerged from her traumatized life.

In her 1960 autobiography *You Learn by Living*, she succinctly sums up her own view of how to transcend the wounds of living: "You gain strength, courage, and confidence by every experience in which you really stop to look fear in the face. . . . You must do the thing you think you cannot do" (Roosevelt, 1960, pp. 29–30).

MARGARET SANGER (1879–1966)

It was the initial wounding precipitated by her mother's 18 pregnancies that influenced the mission of Margaret Sanger to improve the plight of women and fight for birth control. Born Margaret Louise Higgins in Corning, New York, she and her siblings often had to fend for themselves because their mother was ill with tuberculosis and eventually died at the age of forty-nine. The loss of Anne Higgins proved to be a painful wound for young Margaret, a rebellious and independent child. Her alcoholic father also profoundly influenced her with his free-thinking ideas, some of which may have helped her to cope with the early trauma. Although the family had little material wealth, they valued helping others. Her father taught Margaret to "give society the benefit of her honest experience," which was consistent with the family's belief in spite of their poverty (Sanger, 1938, p. 23).

After entering the nursing program at the White Plains Hospital School of Nursing, her probationary period was fraught with traumatic experiences, overexertion, and exhaustion, which resulted in her developing painful, swollen tubercular glands that had to be removed by surgery (Topalian, 1984). After the procedure, the bandage on her right shoulder created a hardship since she had to use her left hand to accomplish most tasks. Another unpleasant event occurred during training when she was attacked by a violent patient suffering from delirium tremens (Topalian, 1984).

These negative experiences diminished in intensity while caring for obstetrical patients, and her new duties made Margaret aware of how completely the women trusted nurses. The exposure greatly stimulated her interest in birth control after delivery, but the indifferent reactions of nurses and physicians to patients' inquiries for more information distressed her in light of the numerous miscarriages and complications.

In 1900, after marrying William Sanger, an architect, Margaret became pregnant and had to be confined temporarily to a sanitarium for treatment of recurring tuberculosis. With the arrival of two more children, she became restless as a wife and mother and joined the Socialist Party with her husband, leaving suburban life and moving to New York City (Bullough, Church, & Stein, 1988).

While practicing home nursing, Margaret Sanger observed firsthand the problems faced by poor working class families. Before long she became their advocate and testified before Congress regarding the abhorrent conditions of women and children in the labor force. She crystallized many of her ideas during this period, believing that reforms regarding women's rights were even more important than the changes needed in wages (Bullough, Church, & Stein, 1988). Committed to this goal, she focused her nursing practice on women's health and published a provocative newspaper column on sex education titled, *What Every Girl Should Know*, which censors of the day immediately attacked as obscene (Katz, 2000).

A significant event in her life took place on a home visit while nursing a woman named Sadie Sachs. The thirty-year-old patient, suffering from septicemia as a result of an unsafe abortion, already had three children and did not wish to become pregnant again. Having been close to death from the procedure, Sadie requested birth control information, which could not be provided legally. Unfortunately, she became pregnant again and after a second self-induced abortion, died in Margaret's presence. This sad event became a turning point for Sanger, who vowed to change the system. The following day, she launched what was to become her courageous cause:

I went to bed knowing what it might cost. I was finished with the pallia-
tives and the superficial cures. I was resolved to seek out the root of
evil, to do something to change the destinies of mothers whose mis-
eries were vast as the skies. (Sanger, 1938, p. 92)

Her mission began with learning about various contraceptive methods and
disseminating information about them. She traveled to France in 1913, meeting with various experts on the subject including the writer Havelock Ellis, an
emerging authority on human sexuality. Upon her return to the United States
a year later, she continued her crusade by challenging the Comstock Law of
1873 that forbade the distribution of birth control information.

In her eight-page monthly newspaper, The Woman Rebel, which first coined
the term "birth control," she aimed to rally support for uniting women against
class and gender oppression. She also prepared a 16-page pamphlet entitled
Family Limitation, which provided explicit instructions for using a variety of contraceptive methods (Katz, 2000). Since these publications included forbidden
information needed by women, Sanger was admonished to cease distribution
immediately. In defying the authorities, she was indicted for violating ob-
scenity laws and faced a sentence of 45 years in prison (Gale Group, 1996).

Shattered by this harsh action but still dedicated to her goal, she fled to
Europe to avoid the legal problems. While there, she found concurrence on
her views relating to sexual liberation for women along with participating
herself in some affairs of the heart. Having divorced Sanger, she later married James L. Slee, an oil magnate, who helped fund her activities in the
birth control movement.

As a true wounded healer, she finally decided to return to the United States
and confront the charges made against her because it was the only way to draw
public attention to her cause. On the eve of the trial in January 1916, however,
trauma struck again when pneumonia suddenly claimed the life of Sanger's
five-year-old daughter. Although her friends and family feared for her health,
she persevered and faced her responsibility to stand up for what she believed
regardless of the consequences. The publicity regarding her child's death, in
addition to the support for the controversial issue of birth control, drew an
outpouring of public empathy that led to the dismissal of the case (Lader &
Meltzer, 1969).

Through her efforts, which included the opening of numerous birth control clinics and eventually the establishment of the International Planned
Parenthood Association, information regarding contraception became available to women worldwide, thus preventing many unnecessary deaths. By
transcending her own trauma, which began with the circumstances of her
mother's life and death, Margaret Sanger took monumental risks and suffered the pain of trying to help other women receive the information they
desperately needed. The year before her death in 1965, the U.S. Supreme
Court handed down its historic decision making birth control legal for married couples (Katz, et al., 2000).

The following compelling words sum up her commitment:

The Revolution came, but not as it had been pictured, nor as history relates that revolutions have come. It came in my own life. It came in my very being. . . . I would strike out—I would scream from the house-tops. I would tell the world what was going on in the lives of these poor women. I would be heard. No matter what it would cost I would be heard! (Topalian, 1984, p. 40)

WILLIAM (BILL) GRIFFITH WILSON (1895–1971)
LOIS BURNHAM WILSON (1891–1988)

Bill and Lois Wilson are perhaps two of the most outstanding examples of wounded healers who have affected the lives of millions of people all over the world. As the cofounders of Alcoholics Anonymous (AA) and Al-Anon, they introduced the 12-step model that became the prototype for the self-help movement launched in the 1970s. Although statistics were never formally maintained on these associations because of member anonymity, the attendance at meetings attested to the higher success rate attained in helping people recover from addiction than from all other methods combined.

The writer Aldous Huxley referred to William Griffith Wilson as the "greatest social architect of the twentieth century" in having saved and changed the lives of countless numbers of people through his vision and work with Alcoholics Anonymous along with Dr. Bob Smith (Steppingstones Foundation, 1999, p. 1). Born and bred in Vermont, Wilson endured an early trauma resulting from the desertion of his alcoholic father who moved to Canada. When he was eleven years old, his parents were divorced, followed by his mother's leaving him and his sister with her parents to pursue medical studies in Boston. Wilson not only suffered from trauma of the parental breakup but also from feelings of severe abandonment.

The good fortune of having loving grandparents, however, helped heal the boy's wounds to some extent. He became an outstanding student, excelled athletically in high school, and taught himself to play the violin. During that time, however, a tragic event occurred when his high school sweetheart, Bertha Bamford, a minister's daughter, died suddenly following a routine surgical procedure. The loss affected Wilson so deeply that he could not complete high school and sank into a serious depression that lasted three years (Steppingstones Foundation, 1999). Although he eventually obtained his diploma, Bertha's sudden death continued to haunt him. In college his grades became erratic because he suffered from anxiety attacks, inferiority feelings, and a lack of self-acceptance (Steppingstones Foundation, 1999).

In 1918, Wilson married Lois Burnham, four years his senior and the daughter of a prominent Brooklyn physician. The oldest of six siblings, she had had a happy childhood with affectionate parents. In later years, she recalls not "wanting to grow up," wishing to remain protected in the loving family environment (Wilson, 1979, p. 1). She attended some of the most prestigious schools, took singing and dancing lessons in her early years, and played basketball in high school. After graduating, she obtained employment as a secretary.

When first meeting Wilson through her brother, Lois did not seem too interested in him but in time the relationship grew and culminated in marriage just before he left to serve in World War I. Although aware of his father's alcoholism, Second Lieutenant Wilson failed to heed his family's warnings to abstain from drinking. Instead, he became addicted to alcohol in the army, claiming that he had "found the elixir of life" (Cheever, 2000, p. 1).

Continuing the habit in civilian life significantly interfered with his law studies. Bill remembered nearly failing some of the courses because he was "too drunk at the finals to think or write," and although he earned his degree, he gave up his goal to practice law (Alcoholics Anonymous, 1976, p. 2). By the time Wilson went on to his next endeavor, as a stockbroker, his wife had already been through several miscarriages. As a result of these traumatic happenings, she was then deprived of her lifelong dream of having children.

As Wilson became more successful in the stock market, his drinking progressed to the stage of putting his stability and resources in jeopardy. Former business associates ostracized him because of his inability to handle alcohol. During the crash of 1929, he lost everything but managed to recover financially. Unfortunately, his successes were reversed rapidly because of the drinking problem, leading to unemployment for at least five years and forcing him and his wife to move in with her parents until their death. At that point, the Wilsons could no longer afford to live in the family home, a big loss to Lois.

At the age of thirty-nine, depleted physically and emotionally, Wilson was admitted twice to a "drying out" hospital in New York. He expressed graphically his revelations of that dark period:

> No words can tell of the loneliness and despair I found in that bitter morass of self-pity. Quicksand stretched around me in all directions, I had met my match, I had been overwhelmed, alcohol was my master. . . . How dark it was before the dawn. (Alcoholics Anonymous, 1976, p. 8)

During his second admission, he claimed to have undergone a spiritual awakening in which he saw a white light and then experienced a sense of acceptance that generated peace (Thomsen, 1975). After his release from the institution, he encountered Ebby, a childhood acquaintance and recovered alcoholic, who told him about the Oxford Group, a spiritual fellowship that had success with helping people stop drinking.

Although Wilson's journey into sobriety took time, he achieved his goal and in 1935 developed the famous 12-step model, assisted by Dr. Bob Smith, also a recovering alcoholic. They based their approach on the principles of the Ox-

ord Group, which included honesty, purity, unselfishness, love, and a belief
n a Higher Power (Steppingstones Foundation, 1996). By then, Wilson had became convinced that by helping other alcoholics, he could save himself.

Lois Wilson also began to transcend her own wounding that had deepened
with her husband's addiction. Unable to dispel the feeling that she had failed
as a woman, which troubled her for years, she recognized the need to exam-
ne her own life (Wilson, 1979, p. 141). Influenced by her husband's recovery,
she acquired new insight as described in her memoirs, *Lois Remembers* (1979):

> After Bill sobered up, it was a great blow for me to realize that he did
> not need me the way he had before. My primary aim in life, helping
> Bill to achieve sobriety had been canceled out, and I had not found
> anything to take its place. Little by little I saw that my ego had been
> nourished during his drinking years by the important roles I had to fill
> as mother, nurse, breadwinner, decision maker. (p. 99) Although sobri-
> ety was what I had been working for all our married life, I had gone
> about it the wrong way. (p. 79)

Realizing that families of alcoholics required support, Lois urged that they
also meet to discuss their concerns and apply the 12-step model of recovery.
Her recommendations paved the way for introducing Al-Anon in 1951. In the
years following what Bill and Lois Wilson presented to society as the most successful treatment program for alcoholism, considerably more has been
learned about addictive disorders. Through the traumatic events in their own
lives, however, these two people found a way to heal themselves and the
wounding of others.

HELEN ADAMS KELLER (1880–1968)
ANNIE MANSFIELD SULLIVAN MACY (1866–1936)

The lives of Helen Adams Keller and Annie Mansfield Sullivan Macy illustrate
how the wounded healer dynamic can emerge between two people. Keller's
poignant story is that of a normal child, who at the age of a year and a half was
shut off suddenly from the life around her. Against overwhelming odds, she
became one of the world's greatest humanitarians. Her parents were Arthur
Keller, a Southern newspaper editor, and Kate Adams Keller, a cultured
woman of New England heritage. The illness that struck their daughter, most
probably scarlet fever, left her blind, deaf, and mute (Keller, 1902).

As she grew from infancy into childhood, young Helen became wild and un-
ruly. When she approached the age of seven, a dramatic event occurred that
she always remembered as "the most important day of [her] life" (Keller, 1902,
p. 16). Through the sympathetic intervention of Alexander Graham Bell, Annie

Mansfield Sullivan entered the home of the Kellers and from that moment on there began a memorable relationship between the twenty-year-old graduate of the Perkins School for the Blind and her young charge. Annie, who had partially regained her own eyesight through a series of operations, transformed the unmanageable youngster into a responsible human being, stimulating her mind and awakening in her a desire to learn (Harrity & Martin, 1962).

Unlike Keller, Sullivan came from poverty, reared in Feeding Hills Massachusetts, the daughter of an ill-tempered father and a caring mother. Her mother's early death exacerbated an earlier trauma already suffered by Annie because of the ravages of trachoma to her eyes. More wounding followed when she and her brother Jimmy, who was crippled from a tubercular hip, were sent to live in the "poor house" in another part of the state. Her brother's death in the wretched institution profoundly affected Annie, and she was determined to change her life and become educated (Bergman, 2000). Through the patient understanding of the teaching staff at Perkins School for the Blind, she progressed rapidly in the program and graduated as valedictorian of her class in 1886 (Bergman, 2000).

Aware of what it was like to be sensorily impaired, Annie knew how to reach the recalcitrant Helen. Although her methods sometimes disturbed the Kellers, she persevered for the good of the child. She and Helen moved to an isolated cottage on the family property to begin the teaching-learning process, and when Helen turned ten, she indicated a desire to learn how to speak (Harrity & Martin, 1962). She made excellent progress and entered Radcliffe College in 1900 accompanied by Annie, who helped her during the program, painstakingly spelling the books and lectures by placing the letters into her hands (Harrity & Martin, 1962). Helen achieved a bachelor of arts cum laude in 1904, the first deaf-blind person to earn a college degree.

Two years earlier, her writing ability had become apparent when she published her autobiography, *The Story of My Life*. While preparing the manuscript, John Albert Macy, an eminent writer, helped her edit the work, and on May 2, 1905, he wed Annie Sullivan in the living room of the Wrentham, Massachusetts, home that the two women shared. The Macys' marriage ended in 1914 when John went to live in Europe, although they were never legally divorced (American Foundation for the Blind, 2000).

For several years, Helen and "Teacher," as she called Annie, traveled throughout the world, devoted to their mission of helping the handicapped (Harrity & Martin, 1962). Although Keller had a wide range of interests, she never lost focus on the needs of the blind and deaf-blind. She appeared before legislatures, gave lectures, wrote numerous articles and books, and showed by her example what a blind person could accomplish. When the American Foundation for the Blind (AFB) was established in 1921, she had acquired an effective outlet for her efforts and served on the staff as a counselor on national and international relations (American Foundation for the Blind, 2000).

During her lifetime, Keller received distinguished awards from nations worldwide, which are displayed in the Helen Keller Room at the AFB in New

York City. Radcliffe also dedicated the Helen Keller Garden in her honor and a fountain named for Annie Sullivan, who also wrote, lectured, and advocated for the deaf. Particularly rewarding for Helen were the friendships and acquaintances she made with leading personalities of the time. Two friends from her youth, Mark Twain and Henry James expressed what so many others admired about her. Twain noted that "the two most interesting characters of the nineteenth century are Napoleon and Helen Keller," and from James came the tribute, "whatever you were or are you're a blessing" (American Foundation for the Blind, 2000, p. 3).

Although Helen Keller outlived Annie Mansfield Sullivan Macy by three decades, their remarkable relationship endured for years. Whenever Helen spoke before audiences, she always alluded to "Teacher" who had led her into the world of hearing and seeing. Whenever Helen spoke, Annie would look on quietly, full of pride in her pupil (American Foundation for the Blind, 2000). Together, they had come a long way, with both transcending the wounding of an earlier period. Six years before she died, Helen Keller expressed the words that perhaps characterized her as one of the great wounded healers of our time: "I thank God for my handicaps, for through them I have found myself, my life and my work" (Harrity & Martin, 1962, p. 7).

MARY BRECKINRIDGE (1881–1965)

The loss of her own two children became the prime impetus for Mary Breckinridge's pioneering efforts devoted to maternal and child care. Long before her first marriage soon after the turn of the century, she enjoyed a privileged life abroad as the daughter of the American ambassador to Russia. Her heritage was eminent in diplomatic circles with her grandfather serving as the vice president of the United States under James Buchanan (Bullough, Church, & Stein, 1988).

When the family came back to the United States in 1900, Breckinridge wed her first husband, who died suddenly two years later from appendicitis (Bullough, Church, & Stein, 1988). Traumatized by this personal tragedy, she traveled to North Carolina to visit friends, and during her stay, witnessed a young child succumb to diphtheria. The event, which stimulated her interest in nursing, ultimately resulted in graduation from the program at St. Luke's Hospital in New York City.

At the age of thirty-one, she married Henry Ruffner Morrision, a college professor, and subsequently gave birth to a son who died when he was only four years old, following a surgical procedure. Prior to this traumatic loss, she had prematurely delivered a baby girl who died shortly after birth (Frontier Nursing Service, 1978). These stresses on her marriage led to divorce. Deeply wounded, she turned to nursing determined to seek new directions.

Breckinridge began her quest by becoming a volunteer nurse in France during World War I. Exposed to the magnitude of suffering of the lost, starving, and orphaned children, she vowed to do everything in her power to help them. Responding to the inadequate supply of milk, she wrote to her friends in the States requesting goats or the money to buy them in order to feed the youngsters. One day, on her return to headquarters, she found 29 goats waiting for her, and after that, the children never lacked milk again (Fried, 1978). Such actions, as well as organizing a child hygiene clinic and a visiting nurse association in France, merited her the Medaille Reconnaissance Française, one of the country's highest honors (Bullough, Church, & Stein, 1988, p. 46).

Motivated to help children after her exposure to human suffering in the war, Breckinridge was eager to make a difference in her native state of Kentucky. Before returning home, she wrote to her mother expressing her desire: "A decision has come to me and not of myself. . . . I am to work directly for little children now, and for always because that is the work I can do best, in which my health, enthusiasm and happiness do not fail" (Breckinridge, 1972, p. 111). After making this pledge, Mary recognized the critical need for good obstetrical care and children's health services in the rural areas of the state, aware that women usually delivered their babies in unsafe and unsterile conditions (Breckinridge, 1972).

Realizing that she herself required more skills, Breckinridge remembered the work of British nurse midwives during the war and decided to undertake midwifery training in London. After completing the course, her next step was to establish preliminary headquarters in Leslie County, Kentucky, assisted by British nurse midwives whom she had met during her studies abroad (Allen, 2000, p. 1). In 1925, with funds inherited from her mother, Breckinridge helped establish the Kentucky Committee for Mothers and Babies, later renamed the Frontier Nursing Service (FNS), and she continued to raise substantial monies from outside sources to keep the enterprise running.

The mission of the FNS clearly reflected Breckinridge's need to transcend the painful losses of her son and daughter. In her own words, she noted the following: "Work for children should begin before they are born, should carry them through their greatest hazard which is childbirth, and should be most intensive during their first six years of life. These are the formative years" (Breckinridge, 1972, p. 111).

Known as "nurses on horseback," the midwives received their early training in rural Kentucky and traveled under perilous conditions, providing patients with adequate prenatal and obstetrical care and treating dietary deficiencies and parasitic infections. With their specially designed saddlebags loaded with needed supplies, these committed professionals ministered to large, destitute families living in primitive houses (Allen, 2000). Breckinridge and her colleagues would often remain overnight with their patients to ensure that both mother and baby remained in stable condition.

Although the technology of the modern information age has produced changes in the way maternal and child care is delivered, the Frontier Nursing Service has remained steadfast in its purpose. Its endurance stands as a gacy to Mary Breckinridge and the enormous contribution she made by her bility to transcend the hurtful events of her earlier years and improve the ealth care of families.

THE CONTEMPORARY HEALER

Undoubtedly, modern society abounds with people whom we may identify s true wounded healers. How many human beings are there who have not xperienced some sort of trauma in their lives? How many have gone on to ranscend their woundedness and heal themselves? And more signifiantly, how many have developed the capacity and skill to facilitate healng in others?

Perhaps no individual exemplifies the wounded healer of today more than Nelson Rolihlahla Mandela, a courageous and remarkable man who overcame decades of wounding and emerged to heal an entire nation. Here is his story.

Nelson Rolihlahla Mandela

During the formative period in his life, Rolihlahla Mandela lived with his family in an isolated provincial village near the shores of the Indian Ocean in the Transkei region of South Africa. After his father's premature death, the Thembu Chief raised the boy to assume an important place in the tribal community, where he learned about the aggression of foreign settlers and determined to dedicate his life to the search for freedom.

After completing his early education in a missionary school, where a teacher arbitrarily changed his name to Nelson, the boy was sent away to an elite institution, the Healdtown Methodist Boarding School. Yet, it was not until he went to Johannesburg in 1941 that Mandela became exposed to racial injustice and its traumatic aftermath.

Although shy and reluctant to speak in public because of his poor English, he overcame the problem, eventually became a lawyer, and opened the first black law firm in the country. Politically active, he headed the African National Congress (ANC), a grass roots organization committed to the self-determination of his people. When apartheid, a policy of strict racial segregation and discrimination was instituted in 1948, Mandela, like Gandhi before him, launched a campaign of defiance through civil disobedience.

The approach he used, however, dramatically changed after a group of 69 black demonstrators were massacred at Sharpeville in 1960, and Mandela organized a paramilitary group to engage in guerrilla warfare against the government. To accomplish his aims, he literally went "underground" for months to alter the mission of the ANC from passive resistance to active engagement, using the term "spear of the nation" to describe the formerly peaceful organization (Arts & Entertainment, 1997). At this point, he fled to Ethiopia and Algeria to undergo military training and from there went to London to study and prepare himself for the difficulties to come.

Returning to South Africa, he received a 5-year prison sentence for inciting a strike and leaving the country illegally in 1962. Two years following his incarceration, he was charged with sabotage and conspiring to overthrow the government, which increased his sentence to life imprisonment. Regarding the trial as "the last chance to show the world the pain and suffering" of South Africa, Mandela and his compatriots pleaded guilty to the charges and refused to defend themselves even when facing the death penalty (Arts & Entertainment, 1997). This response was an attempt to reveal that although the men had been complicit in the acts for which they were indicted, the apartheid government was the real culprit because of the atrocities it inflicted on the people.

At the conclusion of the trial, Mandela's words illustrated the core convictions that directed his life:

> I have fought against white domination and I have fought against black domination. I have cherished the ideal of a democratic and free society in which all persons live together in harmony and with equal opportunities. It is an ideal for which I hope to live for and to achieve, but if needs be, it is an ideal for I am prepared to die. (Arts & Entertainment, 1997).

His greatest wounding followed when he was remanded to Robben Island, a prison similar to Alcatraz, located seven miles off the coast of South Africa, and completely cut off from civilization. There, he underwent severe deprivation of the basic necessities, such as clothing and food, and was subjected to the punishment of laboring in a rock quarry under the blazing hot African sun, oftentimes with inadequate covering to protect himself.

In spite of what seemed like inhumane conditions, his spirits remained high and generated respect from the other prisoners. He even earned admiration from his captors whom he forgave, and who permitted him to organize political education classes. The 30-year ordeal involved a painful separation from his family, but he transformed the circumstances of his fate into a more positive experience. Another traumatic event occurred, however, when his oldest son died in an automobile crash, and he was prohibited from attending the funeral, "leaving a hole in his heart that could never be filled" (A&E, 1997).

Mandela's deliverance from the restrictions and isolation of prison life occurred on his release at the age of seventy-one. As a person of great fortitude and conviction, he had learned to transcend his woundedness because of his faith in being "bigger than it all" and dispelling any bitterness (A&E, 1997). In 1993, he shared the Nobel Peace prize with South African President F. W. deKlerk for their efforts to eliminate apartheid. In the following year, he became the president of a new South Africa in the nation's first free election. During his term, important changes included the provision of free health care for pregnant women and a free lunch daily for each school child.

Although he retired from the presidency in 1999, Nelson Mandela has continued to symbolize the wounded healer in a liberated but still troubled society. He represents a powerful role model, demonstrating that healing can be

TABLE 8–1   ON BECOMING A WOUNDED HEALER

ngeles Arrien (1993), an expert on the culture of indigenous peoples, noted hat the path of the healer involves attention to what has worth and neaning. To help you gain insight as you undertake your quest, reflect on he following core values associated with the wounded healer vignettes.

Ayla: Beyond survival to identity

Hana: Releasing control

Margaret Houlihan: Ongoing growth and development

Celie: Integrating trauma

George Bailey: True self-worth

Lord Jim: Integrity

Randall P. McMurphy: Altruism

Judah Ben Hur: Determination

John Coffey: Love

Harriet Tubman: Perseverance

Margaret Sanger: Courage of one's convictions

Eleanor Roosevelt: Self-acceptance

Nelson Mandela: Forgiveness

Bill and Lois Wilson: Trailblazing

Hellen Keller and Annie Sullivan: Overcoming handicaps/Accepting limitations

Mary Breckinridge: Resolving Grief

Carl Jung: Vulnerability

Arrien, A. (1993). The Four-fold way: Walking the path of the warrior, teacher, healer and visionary. San Francisco: Harper.

achieved with an ability to overcome obstacles and convert them into heroic acts. In his inaugural address on May 10, 1994, he revealed some moving thoughts about the experience of self-transcendence:

> We are born to make manifest the Glory of God that is within us. It's not just in some of us, it's in everyone, and, as we let our light shine, we consciously give other people permission to do the same. As we are liberated from our own fear, our presence automatically liberates others. (Mandela, 1994, p. 540)

REFERENCES

Art & Entertainment Television Network (1994). *Eleanor Roosevelt: A restless spirit*. [Video-cassette]. Available: New Video Group, 126 Fifth Avenue, New York, N.Y., 10011.

Arts & Entertainment Television Network (1997). *Nelson Mandela: Journey to freedom* [Video-cassette]. Available: New Video Group, 126 Fifth Avenue, New York, N.Y., 10011.

Arts & Entertainment Television Network (2000). *Eleanor Roosevelt*. Biography Online Database. http://www.biography.com/find/find.html.

Alcoholics Anonymous (1976). *Alcoholics Anonymous: The story of how many thousands of men and women have recovered from alcoholism* (3rd ed.). New York: Alcoholics Anonymous World Services.

Allen, S. (2000). History of the Frontier Nursing Service. *The Frontier Nursing Service Oral History Project* [Online]. http://www.uky.edu /Libraries/Special/ oral __history/fns.html.

American Foundation for the Blind (2000). *The life of Helen Keller*. afbinfo@afb.net.

Arrien, A. (1993). *The four-fold way: Walking the path of the warrior, teacher, healer and visionary*. San Francisco: Harper.

Bergman, A. (2000). *Annie Mansfield Sullivan Macy: Helen Keller's teacher*. New York: American Foundation for the Blind [Online] http://www.afb.org.

Boeree, G. (1997). *History of psychology: Personality theories: Carl Jung*. www.ship.edu/~ cgboeree/jung.html.

Bradford, S. (1993). *Harriet Tubman: The Moses of her people*. Bedford, MA: Applewood. (Original work published 1886)

Breckinridge, M., 1972. *Wide neighborhood: A story of the Frontier Nursing Service*. New York: Harper.

Brewer, K. (1978). Harriet Tubman: The Moses of her people. *American Nurse*, 10 (5), p. 2.

Bullough, V. L., Church, O. M., & Stein, A. (1988). *American nursing: A biographical dictionary*. New York: Garland.

Cheever, S. (2000). *The Healer Bill Wilson*. Time 100: Heroes & Icons. http://www.pathfinders.com/time/time100/.

Cook, E. (1913). *The Life of Florence Nightingale* (Vol. II). London: Macmillan.

Dunne, C. (2000). *Carl Jung: Wounded healer of the soul*. New York: Parabola.

Encyclopedia Americana (2000). *The American presidency: Eleanor Roosevelt* [Online]. Grolier Inc.

Fowler, E. (1978). Nursing pays tribute to Harriet Tubman. *American Nurse*, 10, (5), p. 1

Fried, J. (1978). Frontier Nursing Service Collection: An interview with Betty Lester. University of Kentucky Oral History Program [Online]. http://www.uky.edu / Libraries/Special/oral __history/fns.html.

Frontier Nursing Service. (1978). University of Kentucky Oral History Program [Online]. http://www.uky.edu /Libraries/Special/oral __history/fns.html.

Gale Group, Inc. (1996). Margaret Sanger. U.X.L® *Biographies* [Online]

Harbart, K., & Hunsinger, M. (1991). The impact of traumatic stress reactions on caregivers. *The Journal of the American Academy of Physicians Assistants*, 4 (5), 384–394.

Harriet Tubman Home (2000). *The life of Harriet Tubman*. HThome@localnet.com.

Harrity, R., & Martin, R. G. (1962). *The three lives of Helen Keller*. Garden City, NY: Doubleday.

Jung, C. G. (1929). Problems of modern psychotherapy. In H. Read, M. Fordham, G. Adler, & W. McGuire (Eds.), *The collected works of* C. G. Jung (CW 16). Princeton, NJ: Princeton University Press.

Jung, C. G. (1989). *Memories, dreams and reflections*. New York: Vintage. (Original work published 1963).

Katz, E., et al. (2000). *The papers of Margaret Sanger* (Columbia, SC: Model Editions Partnership, 1999) Electronic version. http://adh.sc.edu.

Keller, H. (1902). *Helen Keller: The story of my life.* New York: Signet.

Lader, L., & Meltzer, M. (1969). *Margaret Sanger: Pioneer of birth control.* New York: Crowell.

Mandela, N. (1994). *The long walk to freedom.* New York: Little, Brown.

McLynn, F. (1996). *Carl Gustav Jung.* New York: St. Martin's Press.

Micrsoft® Encarta® Online Encyclopedia (2000). *Eleanor Roosevelt.*

Montgomery-Dossey, B. M. (1998). Florence Nightingale: Her Crimean fever and chronic illness. *Journal of Holistic Nursing, 16* (2), 168–196.

Montgomery-Dossey, B. M. (2000). *Florence Nightingale: Mystic, visionary, healer.* Springhouse, PA: Springhouse.

Roosevelt, E. (1960). *You learn by living.* Westminster: Knox.

Sahlman, R. (2000). Harriet Tubman. *Spectrum Home and School Magazine.* [http://www.incwell.com/Spectrum.html] © Inc.Well DMG. Ltd.

Sanger, M. (1938). *Margaret Sanger: An autobiography.* New York: Norton.

Selanders, L. C. (1998). Florence Nightingale: The social impact of feminist values nursing. *Journal of Holistic Nursing, 16* (2), 227–243.

Siegel, B. (1991). *Faithful friend: The story of Florence Nightingale.* New York: Scholastic.

Steppingstones, Foundation (1999) *Bill and Lois' Story.* http://wwwsteppingstones.org/.

Sterling, P., & Logan, R. (1967). *Four took freedom.* New York: Zenith.

Thomsen, R. (1975). *Bill W.* New York: Harper & Row.

Topalian, E. (1984). *Margaret Sanger.* New York: Watts.

Wiesen-Cook, B. (1992). *Eleanor Roosevelt, Vol. 1: 1884–1932.* New York: Viking Penguin.

Wilson, L. (1979). *Lois remembers: Memoirs of the co-founder of Al-Anon and wife of the co-founder of Alcoholics Anonymous.* Virginia Beach, VA: Al-Anon Family Group Headquarters.

CHAPTER 9

PROSPECTS FOR THE FUTURE: WOUNDING AND HEALING

The wounded healer is not an individual once wounded, now recovered, but one who remains vulnerable as well.

David Sedgwick, *The Wounded Healer:*
Countertransference from a Jungian Perspective

Marked variations in past and present healing environments will undoubtedly affect the future of caregiving practices. Although the potential for wounding is ever present as part of the human condition, traumatic episodes can be increasingly resolved and do not necessarily have to remain locked away in anticipation of their disappearing forever or being forgotten. Untreated trauma regardless of its duration has a way of surfacing, with its manifestations revealed through repetitive patterns, addictions, and even what might appear as innocuous or inconsequential habits.

Until the 1970s, the definition of trauma was associated primarily with physiological manifestations because most people were reluctant to share their inner emotional woundedness, particularly when conscious of it. Also, a diagnosis of posttraumatic stress disorder seemed to be reserved for war veterans or victims of natural disasters. Further, society lacked the appropriate role models for generating effective dialogue that would uncover painful events.

At the outset of the twenty-first century, we may question what kinds of trauma will predominate in the coming years, particularly in a global society where technology will continue to advance along with science. At present, the incidence of violence and its graphic portrayal in the media have already desensitized members of society to its dire repercussions. In recent years, barbaric happenings at schools and places of employment as well as acts of cruelty against small children have left the public stunned. We can only wonder if people with serious emotional disorders will seek healing solutions or continue to inflict woundedness on others by their antisocial and unacceptable behavior.

The rise of worldwide terrorism represents a form of trauma that has become inherent within societal consciousness. Our nation has realized its vulnerability to such heinous occurrences as the bombings of the World Trade Center and the Federal Building in Oklahoma City. A deeply embedded fear of potential violence can leave a traumatic residue that remains undetected. Although it may not seem particularly desirable to dwell on the prevalence of trauma, finding solutions for prevention and healing can best be accomplished by facing reality rather than repressing it.

Not all examples have to be as extreme as those cited, since the impact of more subtle forms of wounding can be just as detrimental. Reflect for a moment on the different addictions in the general population. More common than generally believed are such conditions as anorexia and bulimia, which occur in young girls obsessed with being thin. On the other hand, what about the pervasive obesity caused by compulsive or improper eating?

Gambling, as another behavioral problem, not only takes place in casinos but in the form of daily and weekly lotteries. Alcoholism and drug abuse are still rampant, while workaholism appears to flourish among high-powered executives as well as individuals in less prominent types of employment, who perhaps spend unnecessary time on the job to escape from certain realities in their lives.

Included among the newer addictions, and intensifying rapidly, is the use of electronic communication. This medium offers so many attractive features that we often wonder how we managed without it. Yet, certain abuses are not unusual, such as compulsive stock trading and the addiction of children to games, cartoons, and inappropriate programming online. Equally destructive has been the excessive amount of attention that many people devote to television mediocrity, limiting the time for interaction that is conducive to forming healthy relationships with family and friends. And what about the detachment, or "tuning out," that can occur when people walk around with headphones, as well as the potential for reduced hearing—an unrecognized trauma from listening to loud music.

Behavioral illnesses such as addictions often represent attempts to cover up pain or feelings of inadequacy. In some respects, we can point to society as the culprit. The familial disconnections that may occur when couples divorce or when a single parent must work outside the home to support the household can lead to feelings of alienation, anger, and an inability to achieve intimacy (Wallerstein, Lewis, & Blakeslee, 2000). Everyday situations exist in which people retreat from accepted values and adopt less conventional lifestyles to acquire a greater sense of independence and freedom. Yet, unless they demonstrate the responsibility concomitant with nontraditional arrangements, hurtful scars can occur.

Another disheartening issue concerns the pattern of overachievement that becomes addictive when parents urge their offspring to participate in an excessive number of outside recreational activities. What about all those scheduled music and dancing lessons, athletic activities, scouting, and other forms

f structured programming? Undoubtedly, some of these pastimes can gen-
rate positive outcomes such as encouraging team participation and enhanc-
ng social skills. On the other hand, disproportionate involvement, or
busyness," can make children into robots, preventing them from growing nat-
rally, developing internal resources, and establishing strong bonds with their
peers and families. The potential for wounding early in life can be consider-
bly lessened by supporting a youngster's natural inclination toward individ-
ality and seeking creative outlets of his or her liking.

Political differences prominent in the election of government officials may
also create a traumatic aftermath. When the results appear close or uncertain,
not only does cynicism arise among the candidates, but the public becomes
frustrated when healing cannot take place with all the parties involved.

THE HEALING JOURNEY

The wounded healer's story is often equated with the journey of the hero or
heroine who returns home to gather the strength to face the quest ahead. This
excursion may not necessarily require physical travel, but rather a spiritual
awakening that usually evolves after a traumatic event. Consider Mary Breckinridge resettling in rural Kentucky to initiate the Frontier Nursing Service after losing her children, or Harriet Tubman traveling to the South numerous
times under dangerous circumstances to develop the Underground Railroad.
And what of the struggle of Celie whose homecoming provided healing for her
entire family, or Nelson Mandela who emerged from exile to heal a nation.

The ability to surmount life's obstacles never ceases, with many sojourns
into our own personal sanctuary. We may emerge from them with a sense of
relief and a healed vision for the future, or we may endure an inner darkness
that pervades for long periods, which makes it difficult to project a brighter future. Surviving trauma involves confronting the problem, identifying the
source, and reclaiming the inner spirit.

The nursing profession must also search for appropriate ways to foster healing. Although it can claim marked growth in defining the discipline and in raising education and practice standards, it continues to experience severe
wounding in other areas. The resolution of old and deep-seated problems begins with a recognition of the contributing forces. Implicit in this awakening is
that health professionals understand their own vulnerability as a key issue in
dealing with traumatic situations.

As a normal human emotion, human vulnerability may be a form of anxiety that stems from our consciousness, separateness, and mortality (Schaub
& Schaub, 1997). No one wants to appear vulnerable, and in wounded individuals the attempt to cover up their trauma becomes even more essential
as they strive to prevent further insult. We may question why caring people,
especially nurses, seem to have this proclivity toward wounding. Is it because nursing itself may be a metaphor for vulnerability? (Fagin & Diers,

1983). After all, practitioners become exposed to the most intimate of situations when caring for the sick.

As nurses, we often must contend with feelings difficult to process. One unfortunate outcome may be resorting to maladaptive behaviors such as *horizontal violence*, which results in the mistreatment of other colleagues. When oppressed individuals believe that they are helpless to oppose the dominant powerful social group, their thwarted aggression may be inflicted on one another, thus spreading the wounding (Freire, 2000). Nurses have acknowledged this phenomenon when they proclaim that the profession "eats its young" or that they are "the walking wounded." Instead of promoting useful insights to further productive change, such expressions regrettably persist as nothing more than meaningless clichés.

What then might be viewed as the profession's passport to recovery? Feelings of vulnerability must be accepted without shame or guilt, and we must encourage other nurses to join in the healing process and return vigorously to nursing's core values of caring, compassion, and empathy. Without these virtues, how can we hope to transcend the trauma and claim our true identity?

When the foundation of personal and professional healing has been initiated, nursing must persevere with other steps to improve its status internally as well as in the larger society. Some of these factors include elevating education to its highest levels, performing significant research, improving clinical practice, and ensuring our own autonomy and self-regulation.

The act of transcending involves a tedious but thoughtful adventure with rewards that far surpass any unresolved trauma. Healers must be willing to submit to the "dark night" so that they can emerge into the light. What a glorious expectation for nurses to be armed with the knowledge that they are wounded healers who have participated in transforming their own health and that of others. In exploring wounding in the profession, isn't it time, therefore, that we begin our quest with newly acquired strength and a willingness to effect change?

REFERENCES

Fagin, C., & Diers, D. (1983). Nursing as metaphor. *New England Journal of Medicine, 309* (2), 116–117

Freire, P. (2000). *Pedagogy of the oppressed.* New York: Continuum International. (Original work published 1970)

Schaub, B., & Schaub, R. (1997). *Healing addictions.* Albany: Delmar.

Sedgwick, D. (1994). *The wounded healer: Countertransference from a Jungian perspective.* London: Routeledge.

Wallerstein, J., Lewis, J., & Blakeslee, S. (2000). *The unexpected legacy of divorce.* Burbank, CA: Hyperion.

APPENDIX

THE Q.U.E.S.T. MODEL: TRANSCENDING TRAUMA

Phenomenological investigations and clinical practice patterns are the theoretical bases for the Q.U.E.S.T. model for transcending trauma, along with professional experiences, the trauma literature, and other models of reflective practice. Themes related to traumatic episodes that apply to the wounded healer have emerged from research on the therapeutic use of self. A significant observation is that personal trauma becomes a prime factor in nursing, particularly in the care of individuals suffering severe physiological and emotional woundedness.

Predominant among the themes generated from various studies is the ability to *empathize with patients through shared trauma and recovery*, which can be affected in both positive and negative ways. Also prominent are *recognizing and experiencing the manifestation of a mutual trauma, neutralizing mutual trauma through reflection, connecting with while separating from the patient*, and *continued self-development, transformation, and transcendence through therapeutic use of trauma*.

Several assumptions underlying the Q.U.E.S.T. model are identified as follows:

1. Growth and transcendence are an unending process.
2. Trauma patterns, such as parentification, may appear more commonly than realized within all types of relationships.
3. Recovery begins only when nurses and other caregivers remain open to the possibility of trauma occurring in their lives.
4. Transformation and transcendence become possible through understanding the pain caused by trauma, both personally and professionally.
5. Therapeutic use of self can be facilitated when practitioners consciously and deliberately apply their knowledge of trauma to foster mutual growth between themselves and their patients.

THE MODEL

The goal of the Q.U.E.S.T. model is to assist nurses and other health professionals in healing themselves and their profession, and at the same time to avoid vicarious retraumatization in the workplace. Saakvitne & Pearlman (1996) identify several major influences on this phenomenon, including feelings of hopelessness, plus family history and employment setting. The consequences are similar to posttraumatic stress disorder revealing such symptoms as anxiety, depression, intrusive thoughts, alienation, dissociative episodes, and despair. Also noted have been paranoia, hypervigilance, disrupted personal relationships, psychic numbing, and a sense of being overwhelmed (Blair & Ramones, 1996; Saakvitne & Pearlman, 1996).

The steps in the Q.U.E.S.T model include:

Question

Uncover

Experience

Search for Meaning

Transform

Transcend

Question

The act of questioning assumes a form of self-examination that may not come easily to you. Begin by exploring the possibility of having experienced some trauma in your life as well as its subsequent impact. This type of inquiry can be triggered by certain events in the work environment.

In such cases, be willing to raise questions regarding your own personal situation and the potential injury reinforced in clinical practice when caring for patients. Preparing for change leading to transformation requires that you perform a self-assessment as the first step in facing potentially painful revelations that may surface. Otherwise, unhealed trauma contributes to present and future illnesses within the body-mind and counteracts a healing environment.

When initiating the questioning process, determine initially whether you could be among the walking wounded or on the way to becoming a wounded healer (see Table A–1). Try to provide your answers as honestly as possible without allowing the results to become too upsetting. View the activity as an exploratory exercise and a tool for increasing self-awareness.

If addictive or dysfunctional behaviors are present in your life, they can indicate the possibility of some deeply ingrained traumatic pattern. Such observations can be difficult to accept because whatever the conduct, it acts as a defense against the pain. Keep in mind that for recovery to begin, the dis-

TABLE A–1 WALKING WOUNDED OR WOUNDED HEALER?

The following self-assessment guide will help you determine how and if trauma has affected your life, and whether you fit the characteristics of "wounded healer" or "walking wounded." Please note that this exercise aims to identify some past or present characteristics of underlying wounding and is neither inclusive nor a substitute for consulting a professional therapist. Study your responses carefully and with expert assistance as needed.

Respond to each question on the scale of 1 to 3, as indicated below. Then total your score and analyze it according to the criteria.

1 = never
2 = sometimes
3 = always

STATEMENT	SCORE
1. I tend to the needs of others before my own.	_____
2. I become angry easily when facing difficult patient care situations.	_____
3. I have difficulty sharing my feelings.	_____
4. I experience unexplained bodily sensations.	_____
5. I believe I have unresolved traumatic experiences in my life.	_____
6. I don't remember many early childhood experiences.	_____
7. I consider leaving the helping profession.	_____
8. I tend to have unexplained, distressing emotional reactions at work.	_____
9. I feel emotionally numb most of the time.	_____
10. I startle easily.	_____
11. I consider seeking psychological counseling.	_____
12. I engage in addictive behaviors (drinking to excess, eating, smoking, or excessive shopping).	_____
13. I have poor relationships with my family.	_____
14. I have disturbing thoughts that I can't seem to control.	_____
15. I avoid people places and things that remind me of the past.	_____
16. I find my work environment stressful.	_____
17. I have vivid, disturbing memories of past events in my life.	_____
18. I have a negative outlook on life.	_____
19. I feel helpless to change my situation.	_____
20. I prefer being alone.	_____

tress of the addiction needs to be greater than that of facing the trauma. A person addicted to alcohol, for example, must realize that the destructive consequences of excessive drinking are more painful than the extreme discomfort that occurs in achieving sobriety. If guidance is needed in helping you resolve your problems, consider self-help groups since they can be quite supportive and an effective resource to begin your quest.

Scoring

0–20: You may not have experienced much trauma in your life, or you may be well on your way to transcending it and becoming a wounded healer. You also may be in denial that trauma has been a part of your life.

21–40: You show warning signals that suggest the surfacing of past trauma, but you may not be aware of the precipitating factors. Consider further self-exploration with peers and/or professionals.

41–60: You have experienced trauma and may be among the walking wounded. Professional guidance is suggested to help alleviate your pain.

Uncover

After the initial questioning, uncovering trauma patterns is the next step and perhaps the one most resisted because of the difficulty in remembering, as well as the concern about potential ramifications of recalling painful memories. If abuse has occurred, especially at the hands of relatives, it may not be possible to deal with them for fear of rejection. Also, the response to trauma can result in self-abuse or mistreating others. In some situations, nurses tend to hurt one another because they feel victimized in the work environment. One of the most common examples occurs when offering unwarranted criticism instead of constructive support.

You should be aware that many common traumas will not be uncovered as a single memory of a specific event. A more beneficial approach to detecting areas of wounding comes from an analysis of behavior patterns. The process requires courage as well as support because of the potential pain that may arise. Therefore, a qualified therapist can help obtain the desired result.

Unfortunately, it becomes counterproductive when the caregiver is a wounded individual with unresolved trauma. There arises a breach of the therapeutic contract when health professionals appear to be working out their own issues within therapeutic relationships. Some telltale signs of this phenomenon exist when they inappropriately share intimate details of their own lives or, at the other extreme, appear to be detached or respond inappropriately to what the patient shares. A willingness to listen to concerns and to

hange personal behavior indicates movement toward growth and self-tran-
cendence for the practitioner. If on the other hand, attempts are made to
place the responsibility solely on the patient's perceptions, another professional should be consulted to avoid retraumatization.

A key element in uncovering trauma depends on the willingness of nurses
to face their own pain. In helping others who have been wounded, one way to
begin may be by examining old photographs of yourself at various points in
your life. If you suspect that a certain incident happened at a specific age,
study a snapshot taken at that time. Try to imagine the feelings of the child in
the photograph as well as what the facial expressions, the dress, and the entire appearance can tell you. Also, who else is in the picture? Jot down your responses in a journal because they can eventually lead to new insights.
Maintaining a record and reflecting on it will help illuminate perceptions for
further introspection.

Experience

This step can be difficult to achieve because wounded persons may not be
able to accept what has happened to them and usually repress certain occurrences. Awareness of an event and experiencing it on an emotional level
cannot be perceived as being identical. Even when an individual harbors a
great degree of cognitive insight, it does not necessarily predict recovery. As
Myss (1997) reminds us, such individuals tend to cling to their own wounds
without being able to process or transcend them. Although such behavior unwittingly may imply that they are addressing the problem, rarely do they go
beyond this phase to accepting their woundedness. The answer, however,
does not lie in attempting to obliterate the traumatic episode from memory
but rather to acquire a fresh perspective on it. The most powerful shamans,
as we may recall, are often recognized by their transcendence of significant
wounding.

Search for Meaning

Why is it important for us to search for the meaning of trauma and its relationship to transcendence? This step can be viewed as the most critical since it
seeks to acquire a perspective that will promote healing. It is desirable to remember that severe wounding changes the perception of the victim who afterward sees the world through the veil of the injury. The seriousness of the
traumatic episode lies within its "timeless nature" (van der Kolk & McFarlene,
1996) and its ability to become frozen within the body-mind (Levine & Frederick, 1997).

In situations where words do not exist to describe the wounding, how then
can an emotional catharsis be effected? It has been demonstrated that art and
literary works can help markedly to tap into our unspoken feelings. Often, a

therapeutic release takes place when people draw or paint images that express deep emotions or even when they observe the contributions of others. Such activities help us find meaning in our suffering and initiate the healing process through an expression of repressed feelings.

Rose (1995) asserts that art communicates different meanings to different people, succeeding where other media fail in healing trauma. The work is "indirect, unaesthesized and dialogic in nature," creating a "witnessing presence" that acts as an antidote to the self-destructiveness of a severely wounded individual (Laub & Podell, 1995, p. 991). A major impediment to transforming and transcending trauma has been the continuing sense of disconnection experienced by the victim. Anyone who has known what it means to feel segregated and isolated from others can understand the chronic pain of the wounded survivor. Searching for and understanding the meaning behind the suffering becomes a necessary aim toward attaining a higher level of consciousness and transcendence.

Transform and Transcend

In the final step, the individual develops the capability for examining past events with renewed awareness. If viewing a specific situation or pattern of behavior in a new way represents the path to transcendence, why is such a desirable goal so difficult to accomplish? A major factor in the process of transforming is to forgive one's self as well as others, which should lead to such outcomes as alleviating shame and discarding the traumatic worldview. Shame, on the other hand, inspires negative thinking and destroys the "interpersonal bridge" between ourselves and others (Kaufman, 1985).

Another way of comprehending the dynamics underlying the nature and effect of trauma is recognizing the "failure of empathy," which prompts individuals to commit antisocial or harmful acts (Laub & Podell, 1995). When caregivers cannot face their own shame or accept the vulnerabilities of others, they continue to be wounded.

In Figure A–1 study the work, *The Door to the Possible*, by Ishmira Kathleen Thoma (1990), whose rich symbolism conveys various impressions to different people. With her head bowed, the woman in the painting appears weary as she emerges from the "waters of life experience," a healing medium (I. K.Thoma, personal communication, December 31, 2000). She can be perceived as the wounded healer ready to transform herself, moving toward an immaterial door with striking symbols of the sun and moon engraved on it. In this illustration, the translucency of the door enables her to see through it to some degree. To the left there are Greek columns that the artist interprets as "past failures," along with mountains in the distance depicting the future to be transcended. A sense of lightness and heaviness emerges simultaneously as the woman trudges through the water carrying what seems to be a heavy emotional burden. Yet, the surroundings seem serene, with hope for transcendence on the horizon.

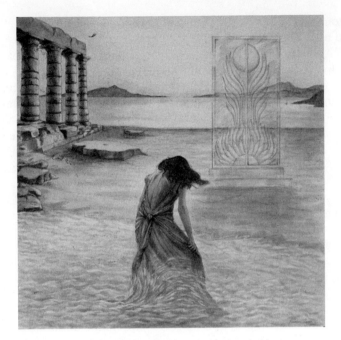

Figure A–1 *The Door to the Possible*, Ishmira Kathleen Thoma 1990.
Reproductions available from StudioK@ma.ultranet.com.

THE Q.U.E.S.T. MODEL IN ACTION

Sally's Story: Journey to Transcendence

A recipient of a master's degree and with over twenty years of nursing experience, Sally practiced on a medical unit for two years before becoming a psychiatric nurse in a substance abuse treatment center. For a long time she was
attracted to this patient population but had only a vague understanding of her
motivation.

Her family background included a mother with a long history of depression
and social phobias, and a workaholic father who used his focus on career to escape coping with his wife's problems. Being codependent, he made excuses
for the woman's lack of functioning and frequently commented, "Mother is not
well." Sally adapted to the dysfunctional family situation by reading novels,
writing poetry, and attempting to isolate herself from parental arguments.
When forced to interact during their sometimes violent altercations, she appeared calm but was inwardly terrified, experiencing severe palpitations. As
the younger of two female siblings, she described herself as the "good child
who never made waves."

After completing a baccalaureate nursing program, Sally married at the age of 22, had two children, and left her husband after five years because he was abusive physically and emotionally. Divorced and a single parent, she returned to live with her parents while attending graduate school part-time and eventually earned her degree. After a time, when reexposed to the continuing dysfunctional family situation, she began to realize that her seemingly calm demeanor had actually been a coverup for an inner fear whenever violent conflict erupted. This insight was brought more sharply into focus by an event that occurred in the clinical setting.

Working one evening on a drug and alcohol unit in a freestanding building, Sally was the only nurse on duty with a census of thirty patients. At 6 P.M., three male patients approached the nursing station urging her to attend an emergency community meeting that they had convened. The men were distressed by the behavior of Joe, another patient, who physically threatened them and acted seductively toward the women. They were concerned that he was becoming high on cocaine especially since he was bragging about his criminal background.

Sally agreed to join the group without any clear plan on how to proceed. Although an inner terror seized her, she succeeded in reassuring the patients and agreed to speak to Joe. When meeting with him later in the nurses' station, Sally quickly explained that she was not accusing him of anything, but for his own safety as well as the others, it would be better to remain overnight in the observation room under supervision. Although extremely upset about the confrontation on the unit, Joe reluctantly agreed and in the morning spoke with the administrative and clinical staff to resolve the matter. The next day, Joe voluntarily left the facility after showing disruptive behavior from drug use while in treatment.

Question

Prior to the episode described above, Sally had always prided herself on remaining calm in a crisis situation, but the aftermath of what happened with Joe created a need for self-examination. She recalled that throughout her nursing career, it was not unusual to be exposed to distressed chemically dependent patients in various practice settings. Her reaction toward the encounter with the group, however, turned out to be markedly different. Her previous pattern had been to act with equanimity while listening to patients' concerns and working on a treatment plan in which they participated. In light of the present situation, she started to question her behavior.

Uncover

Believing that overwork might have contributed to her initial response, Sally decided to confer with Lynn, a nurse psychotherapist, who also happened to specialize in trauma counseling. Sharing her story, she revealed her feelings of being overwhelmed at the time of the clinical encounter. The pa-

ents, she noted were considerably larger than she and had an air of being
a charge. When they invited her to the meeting for which they had appar-
ntly mapped out a strategy for coping with Joe's disturbing behavior, Sally
eferred to herself as being on the verge of panic—a reaction she success-
ully suppressed.

When Lynn encouraged her to ponder the incident carefully, Sally was then
ble to remember how alone she felt at the time and the sense of inadequacy
n handling the situation. As calm as she appeared at the community meeting,
er heart had been pounding and was accompanied by the fear that some vi-
lence might erupt on the patient unit. After assessing the situation, Lynn
ointed out that Sally's reaction at that time came about because of a repressed trauma which could no longer be contained and suggested that the
urse give some thought to this possibility.

Experience

A week after her session with Lynn, Sally began to have panic attacks when she
hought about the nurse therapist's comments. At their next meeting, she re-
alled the violence in her childhood between her parents and the accompanying fear she had experienced. With Lynn's guidance, she began to make
connections and acknowledge that the patients at the treatment center
looked to her for some intervention just as her parents had done. Although
successful in managing the crisis on the unit, the experience reawakened
dormant painful emotions.

Search for Meaning

When Sally started exploring her outward demeanor of tranquillity in responding to the crisis, Lynn helped her recognize the trauma of parentification. The nurse was able to understand that the behavior demonstrated
toward her family became traumatic since she had grown up beyond her years,
carrying too much responsibility for them. As a result, she repeated this pattern of overresponsibility with others, which made her vulnerable in dangerous situations without consciously experiencing appropriate levels of fear.

Sally finally realized that her abusive marriage and return to the parental
home after the divorce had been instrumental in reviving old feelings that
could no longer be repressed, even at work. To effect change in the work environment, however, she had to admit that she enjoyed the sense of power
and control by appearing calm when critical incidents happened. Lynn helped
her understand that this response was necessary for her to survive traumatic
occurrences.

Transform and Transcend

After reaching a certain level of awareness regarding the pivotal episode,
Sally recognized the need to alter the past ways in which she reacted. It was

not an easy transformation because the dysfunctional behavior offered some comfort as well as a means of coping with difficult situations and providing a sense of self-worth. Eventually, she moved out of her parent's home, which for too long had produced the unwholesome climate that created her early wounding.

Toward the latter sessions with Lynn, Sally's awakening tended to make her more insecure and frightened than before and she confessed to feeling as if she were "falling apart." The therapist reassured her by explaining that the response was a natural and healthy reaction that would help her fully examine her painful experiences and how they affected her life.

About a year after the unpleasant event with Joe, Sally was confronted with a similar situation in the same treatment center where a patient threatened violence on the unit. In this case, she immediately notified the security guard on duty, and after formulating a strategy, they intervened together. Although she remained at ease, her action of seeking help indicated that she no longer continued her old pattern of placing herself in dangerous circumstances alone. Traces of fear still existed, but she had no guilt or shame for seeking assistance or not acting independently. Sally now believed that she had reached the stage of transcending her long-standing trauma and could view future situations with greater confidence and hope.

REFERENCES

Blair, D. T., & Ramones, V. (1996). Understanding vicarious traumatization. *Journal of Psychosocial Nursing, 34* (11), 24–34.

Kaufman, G. (1985). *Shame: The power of caring.* Rochester, VT: Schenkman.

Laub, D., & Podell, D. (1995). Art and trauma. *International Journal of Psychoanalysis, 76* (12), 991–1005

Levine, P., & Frederick, A. (1997). *Walking the tiger: Healing trauma.* Berkeley, CA: North Atlantic.

Myss, C. (1997). *Why people don't heal and how they can.* New York: Harmony.

Saakvitne, K. W., & Pearlman, L. A. (1996). *Transforming the pain: A workbook on vicarious trauamtization.* New York: Norton.

Thoma, I. K. (1990). The Door to the Possible. StudioK@ma.ultranet.com

Rose, G. (1995). *Necessary illusion: Art as "witness."* New York: International University Press.

van der Kolk, B., & McFarlane, A. C. (1996). The black hole of trauma. In B. van der Kolk, A. C. McFarlane, & L.Weisaeth (Eds.), *Traumatic stress: The effects of overwhelming experience on mind, body and society* (pp. 3–23). New York: Guilford.

BIBLIOGRAPHY

Arts & Entertainment (A&E) Television Network, (1997). *Nelson Mandela: Journey to freedom* [Videocassette]. Available: New Video Group, 126 Fifth Avenue, New York, N. Y., 10011.

A & E Televison Network, (1994). *Eleanor Roosevelt: A restless spirit* [Videocassette]. Available: New Video Group, 126 Fifth Avenue, New York, N. Y., 10011.

A & E Television Network (2000). *Eleanor Roosevelt* [Biography Online Database]. http://www.biography.com/find/find.html.

Abrahamsen, V. (1997). The goddess and healing: Nursing's heritage from antiquity. *Journal of Holistic Nursing, 15* (1), 9–24.

Achterberg, J. (1988). The wounded healer: Transformational journeys in modern medicine. In G. Doore (Ed.), *Shaman's path: Healing growth and empowerment* (pp. 115–129). Boston: Shambala.

Achterberg, J. (1991). *Woman as healer: A panoramic survey of women from prehistoric times to the present.* Shambala: Boston.

Achterberg, J., & Lawlis, G. F. (1980). *Bridges of the bodymind: Behavioral approaches to health care.* Champaign, IL: Institute for Personality and Ability Testing.

Adams, J. D. (Ed.). (1986). *Transforming leadership: From vision to results.* Alexandria VA: Miles River Press.

Aesoph, L. M. (2000). The basics of homeopathy. *Great life: Your guide to health and well-being, 4,* 39–41.

Alcoholics Anonymous (1976). *Alcoholics Anonymous: The story of how many thousands of men and women have recovered from alcoholism* (3rd ed.). New York: Alcoholics Anonymous World Services.

Allen, S. (2000). *History of the frontier nursing service. The Frontier Nursing Service Oral History Project* [Online]. http://www.uky.edu /Libraries/Special/oral_history/fns.html.

American Foundation for the Blind (2000). *The life of Helen Keller. afbinfo@afb.net*

Andrews, L. (1989). Mirroring the life force. In R. Carlson and B. Shield (Eds.), *Healers on healing* (pp. 42–47). New York: Penguin Putnam.

Apostle-Mitchell, M., & MacDonald, G. (1997). An innovative approach to pain management in critical care: Therapeutic Touch. *CACCN, 8* (3), 19–22.

Arrien, A. (1993). *The four-fold way: Walking the path of the warrior, teacher, healer and visionary.* San Francisco: Harper.

Auel, J. M. (1980). *The clan of the cave bear.* New York: Bantam.

Bach, E. (1931). *Heal thyself: An explanation of the real cause and cure of disease.* Essex, UK: Daniel.

Bach, E. & Wheeler, F. J. (1997). *The Bach Flower Remedies.* New Canaan, CT: Keats.

Bailey, J. (1998). The supervisor's story: From expert to novice. In C. Johns & D. Freshwater, (Eds.), *Transforming nursing through reflective practice* (pp. 194–205). London: Blackwell Science.

Barrett, E. A. M. (1988). Using Rogers' Science of Unitary Human Beings in nursing practice. *Nursing Science Quarterly*, 1, 50–51.

Bedell-Smith, S. (1999). *Diana in search of herself: Portrait of a troubled princess.* New York: Random House.

Beevers, J. (Trans.) (1989). *The autobiography of Saint Thérèse of Lisieux : The Story of a Soul.* New York: Doubleday.

Beinfield, H., & Korngold, L. (1991). *Between heaven and earth: A guide to Chinese medicine.* New York: Ballantine.

Belanger, D. (2000). Nurses and suicide: The risk is real. RN, 63 (10), 61–64.

Bengtsson, O. (1995). Many doors to healing. In. D. Kunz (Ed.), *Spiritual healing: Doctors examine therapeutic touch and other holistic treatments.* Wheaton, IL: Theosophical Publishing.

Benner, P. (1984). *From novice to expert: Excellence and power in clinical nursing practice.* Menlo Park, CA: Addison-Wesley.

Benner, P., & Tanner, C. (1987). How expert nurses use intuition. *American Journal of Nursing*, 1, 23–31.

Bepko, C., & Krestan, J.A. (1985). *The responsibility trap: A blueprint for treating the alcoholic family.* New York: Free Press.

Bergman, A. (2000). *Annie Mansfield Sullivan Macy: Helen Keller's teacher.* New York: American Foundation for the Blind [Online]. http://www.afb.org.

Blair, D. T., & Ramones, V. (1996). Understanding vicarious traumatization. *Journal of Psychosocial Nursing*, 34 (11), 24–34.

Blumhofer, E. W. (1993). *Aimee Semple McPherson: Everybody's sister.* Grand Rapids, MI: Eermans.

Boeree, G. (1997). *History of psychology: Personality theories: Carl Jung.* www.ship.edu/~cgboeree/jung.html

Bowen, M. (1985). *Family therapy in clinical practice.* New York: Aronson.

Bowlby, J. (1977). The making and breaking of afffectional bonds. *British Journal of Psychiatry*, 130, 201–210.

Bradford, S. (1993). *Harriet Tubman: The Moses of her people.* Bedford, MA: Applewood. (Original work published 1886)

Bradshaw, J. (1995). *Family Secrets: What you don't know can hurt you.* New York: Bantam.

Breckinridge, M., (1972). *Wide neigborhood: A story of the Frontier Nursing Service.* New York: Harper.

Brennan, B. A. (1987). *Hands of light: A guide to healing through the human energy field.* New York: Bantam.

Brennan, B. A. (1993). *Light emerging: The journey of personal healing.* New York: Bantam.

Brewer, K. (1978). Harriet Tubman: The Moses of her people. *American Nurse*, 10 (5), p. 2.

Buber, M. (1965). *Between man and man* (R.G. Smith, Trans.). New York: Macmillan. (Original work published 1937)

Buckle, J. (1997). *Clinical aromatherapy in nursing.* London: Arnold.

Bullough, V. L., Church, O. M., & Stein, A. (1988). *American nursing: A biographical dictionary.* New York: Garland.

Buyssen, H. (1996). *Traumatic experiences of nurses: When your profession becomes a nightmare.* London: Kingsley.

Camp, J. (1973). *Magic, myth and medicine.* New York: Taplinger.

Campbell, J. (1990). *The hero with a thousand faces: Myths: Princeton Bollinger Series in world mythology* (Vol. 17). Princeton, NJ: Princeton University Press.

Capra, F. (Producer & Director). (1946). *It's a wonderful life* [Videocassette]. Available: Goodtimes Homevideo, 401 Fifth Avenue, New York, NY, 10016.

Carlson, R., & Shield, B. (1989). *Healers on healing.* New York: Penguin Putnam.

Carroll, L. (1983). *Alice's adventures in Wonderland* New York: Alfred J. Knopf.

Catherall, D. (1992). *Back from the brink: A family guide to overcoming traumatic stress.* New York: Bantam.

Cayeleff, S. E. (1988). Gender, ideology and the water cure movement. In N. Gevitz. (Ed.), *Other healers: Unorthodox medicine in America* (pp. 82–98). Baltimore: Johns Hopkins.

Celani, D. P. (1994). *The illusion of love: Why the battered woman returns to her abuser.* New York: Columbia University Press.

Cheever, S. (2000). *The Healer Bill Wilson.* Time 100: Heroes & Icons. http://www.pathfinders.com/time/time100/.

Chenitz, C. (1989). Managing vulnerability: Nursing treatment for heroin addicts. *Image: Journal of Nursing Scholarship,* 21 (4), 210–214.

Chinn, P. L., & Kramer, M. K. (1991). *Theory and nursing: A systematic approach.* St. Louis: Mosby.

Christian, B. (1998). *Monarch Notes: Alice Walker's The Color Purple.* New York: Simon & Schuster.

Claridge, K. (1992). Reconstructing memories of abuse: A theory based approach. *Psychotherapy,* 29 (2), 243–252.

Colaizzi, P. F. (1978). Psychological research as the phenomenologist views it. In R. S. Valle (Ed.), *Existential-phenomenological alternatives for psychology.* New York: Oxford University Press.

Conrad, J. (1961). *Lord Jim.* New York: Doubleday. (Original work published 1899)

Cook, E. (1913). *The Life of Florence Nightingale* (Vol. II). London: Macmillan.

Conti-O'Hare, M. (1996). A descriptive analysis of the therapeutic use of self with addicted clients in early recovery from the expert nurse's perspective. *Journal of Addictions Nursing,* 8 (3), 80–84.

Conti-O'Hare, M. (1998). Examining the wounded healer archetype: A case study in expert addictions nursing practice. *Journal of the American Psychiatric Nurses Association,* 4 (3), 71–76.

Cooper, J. C. (1978). *An illustrated encyclopaedia of traditional symbols.* London: Thames and Hudson.

Courtois, C. (1988). *Healing the incest wound.* New York: Norton.

Coward, D. (1991). Self-transcendency and emotional well-being in women with advanced breast cancer. *Oncology Nursing Forum, 18,* 162–169.

Crisp, T. (1990). *Dream dictionary.* New York: Dell.

Crawford, G. (1982). The concept of pattern in nursing: Conceptual development and measurement. *Advances in Nursing Science, 5* (1), 1–6.

Crothers, D. (1995). Vicarious traumatization in the work with survivors of childhood trauma. *Journal of Psychosocial Nursing, 33* (4), 9–13.

Daken, E. (1968). *Mrs. Eddy: The biography of a virginal mind.* Gloucester, MA: Smith.

Davidson, P., & Jackson, C. (1985). The nurse as survivor: Delayed post-traumatic stress reaction and cumulative trauma in nursing. *International Journal of Nursing Studies, 22* (1), 1–13.

Doheny, M., Cook, C., & Stopper, M. (1982). *The discipline of nursing: An introduction.* Bowie, MD: Brady.

Dolan, J., Fitzpatrick, M. L., & Herrmann E. K. (1983). *Nursing in society: A historical perspective.* (15th ed.). Philadelphia: Saunders.

Donahue, P. M. (1985). *Nursing: The finest art: An illustrated history.* St. Louis: Mosby.

Doore, G. (Ed.). (1988). *Shaman's path: Healing growth and empowerment.* Boston: Shambala.

Dorot, R. (Ed.). (1997). *Holyland journey.* Ramat Gan, Israel: Doko.

Dossey, L. (1989). *Recovering the soul: A scientific and spiritual search.* New York: Bantam.

Dryden, J. (2000). *The Internet classics archive/The Aeneid by Virgil.* http://classics.mit.edu/Virgil/aeneid.html.

Dunne, C. (2000). *Carl Jung: Wounded healer of the soul.* New York: Parabola.

Early, E. (1993). *The raven's return: The influence of psychological trauma on individuals and culture.* Wilmette, IL.: Chiron.

Ehenreich, B., & English, D. (1973). *Witches, midwives and nurses: A history of women healers.* New York: Feminist Press.

Ellis, A., & Harper, R. (1975). *A new guide to rational living.* North Hollywood, CA: Wilshire.

Encyclopedia Americana (2000). *The American presidency: Eleanor Roosevelt* [Online]. Grolier Inc.

Epstein, D. M. (1993). *Sister Aimee: The life of Aimee Semple McPherson.* New York: Harcourt Brace Jovanovich.

Epstein, D. (1994). *The 12 stages of healing: A network approach to wholeness.* San Rafael, CA: Amber-Allen.

Erikson, E. (1986). *Vital involvement in old age.* New York: Norton.

Erickson, M., & Rossi, E. (1976/1980). Two level communication and microdynamics of trance. In E. Rossi (Ed.), *The collected papers of Milton H. Erickson on hypnosis and suggestion* (pp. 430–451). New York: Irvington.

Estes, J. W. (1985). George Washington and the doctors: Treating America's first superhero. *Medical Heritage, 1*(1), 12–13.

Fagin, C., & Diers, D. (1983). Nursing as metaphor. *New England Journal of Medicine, 309* (2), 116–117.

Fitzpatrick, J. J. (1992). Reflections on Nightingale's perspective of nursing. In F. Nightingale, *Notes on Nursing* (pp. 18–22). Philadelphia: Lippincott.

Flammonde, P. (1999). *The mystic healers: A history of magical medicine*. New York: Scarborough.

Flaskerud, J. H., Halloran, E. J., Janken, J., Lund, M., & Zetterlund, J. (1979). Avoiding and distancing: A decriptive view of nursing. *Nursing Forum*, 18, (2), 158–174.

Fortune, M. (1995). Is nothing sacred? When sex invades the pastoral relationship. In J. C. Gonsiorek (Ed.), *Breach of trust: Sexual exploitation by health care professionals and clergy* (pp. 29–40).Thousand Oaks, CA: Sage.

Fowler, E. (1978). Nursing pays tribute to Harriet Tubman. *American Nurse*, 10, (5), p. 1.

Frankl, V (1963) *Man's search for meaning: An introduction to logotherapy*. New York: Washington Square Press.

Frankl, V. (1966). Self-transcendence as a human phenomenon. *Journal of Humanistic Psychology*, 6, 97–106.

Freire, P. (2000). *Pedagogy of the oppressed*. New York: Continuum International (Original work published 1970)

Fried, J. (1978). Frontier Nursing Service Collection: An interview with Betty Lester. University of Kentucky Oral History Program [Online]. http://www.uky.edu / Libraries/Special/oral_history/fns.html.

Frontier Nursing Service. (1978). University of Kentucky Oral History Program [Online]. http://www.uky.edu /Libraries/Special/oral_history/fns.html.

Gale Group, Inc. (1996). Margaret Sanger. *U.X.L® Biographies* [Online].

Ganim, B. (1998). *Art and healing: Using expressive art to heal the body, mind and spirit*. New York: Three Rivers Press.

Gatto, J. T. (1998). *Monarch Notes: Ken Kesey's One Flew Over The Cuckoo's Nest*. New York: Simon and Schuster.

Gevitz, N. (Ed.). (1988). *Other healers: Unorthodox medicine in America*. Baltimore: Johns Hopkins.

Ghalioungui, P. (1963). *Magic and medical science in ancient Egypt*. London: Hodder and Stoughton.

Goldstein, J. (1983). *The experience of insight: A simple and direct guide to Buddhist meditation*. London: Shambala.

Gonsiorek, J. C. (Ed.).(1995). *Breach of trust: Sexual exploitation by health care professionals and clergy*. Thousand Oaks, CA: Sage.

Gorkin, M. (1987). *The uses of countertransference*. Northvale, NJ: Aranson.

Grey, A. (1990). *Sacred mirrors: The visionary art of Alex Grey*. Rochester, VT: Inner Traditions.

Groesbeck, C. J. The archetypal image of the wounded healer. *The Journal of Analytical Psychology*, 20, 120–145.

Guggenbuhl-Craig, A. (1971). *Power in the helping professions*. New York: Spring.

Haase, J. E., Britt, T., Coward, D. D., Leidy, N. K., & Penn, P. E. (1992). Simultaneous concept analysis of spiritual perspective, hope, acceptance and self-transcendence. *Image*, 24 (2), 141–147.

Hall, J. (1997). Nursing stress: Applying the wisdom of the wounded healer. *Lamp*, 54 (8), 24–25.

Harbart, K., & Hunsinger, M. (1991). The impact of traumatic stress reactions on caregivers. *The Journal of the American Academy of Physicians Assistants*, 4 (5), 384–394.

Harner, M. (1988). What is a shaman? In G. Doore (Ed.), *Shaman's path: Healing, growth and empowerment* (pp. 7–15). Boston: Shambala.

Harner, M. (1990). *The way of the shaman.* San Francisco: Harper.

Harriet Tubman Home. (2000). *The life of Harriet Tubman.* HThome@localnet.com.

Harrity, R., & Martin, R. G. (1962). *The three lives of Helen Keller.* Garden City, NY: Doubleday.

Hay, L. L. (1987). *You can heal your life.* Carson, CA: Hay House.

Heidt, P. (1981a). Scientific research and Therapeutic Touch. In P. Heidt and M. A. Borelli (Eds.), *Therapeutic Touch* (pp. 3–12). New York: Springer.

Heidt, P. (1981b). Effect of Therapeutic Touch on anxiety level of hospitalized patients. *Nursing Research, 30* (1), 32–37.

Herman, J. L. (1992). *Trauma and recovery: The aftermath of violence from domestic abuse to political terror.* New York: Basic Books.

Herman, J. L., & Schatzow, E. (1987). Recovery and verification of childhood sexual trauma. *Psychoanalytic Psychology, 4* (1), 1–14.

Heuerman, T., & Olson, J. (2000). The allegory of Plato's cave. *Self-Help and Psychology Magazine.* http.shpm.com.

Hickey, E. W. (1997). *Serial murderers and their victims* (2nd ed). Belmont, CA: Wadsworth.

Hillegass, C. K. (1973). *Cliff's notes on mythology* Lincoln, NE: Cliffs Notes.

Hollis, J. (1989). The wounded vision. *Quadrant, 22* (2), 25–36.

Horowitz, M. J. (1986). *Stress response syndromes* (2nd ed.). Northvale, NJ: Jason Aronson.

Hover-Kramer, D., Mentgen, J., & Scandrett-Hibdon, S. (1996). *Healing Touch: A resource for health professionals.* Albany, NY: Delmar.

Hover-Kramer, D. (2000). Relationships. In B. M. Dossey, L. Keegan, & C. E. Guzzeta (Eds.), *Holistic nursing: A handbook for practice* (pp. 639–658). Gaithersberg, MD: Aspen.

James, W. (1950). *The principles of psychology* (Vols. 1–2). New York: Kover.

Johns, C. (1995). The value of reflective practice for nursing. *Journal of Clinical Nursing, 4,* 23–30.

Johns, C., & Freshwater, D. (Eds.). (1998). *Transforming nursing through reflective practice.* London: Blackwell Science.

Jung, C. G. (1913). The theory of psychoanalysis. In H. Read, M. Fordham, G. Adler, & W. McGuire (Eds.), *The collected works of C. G. Jung.* (CW4) *Bolligen Series XX.* Princeton: Princeton University Press.

Jung, C. G. (1929). Problems of modern psychotherapy. In H. Read, M. Fordham, G. Adler, & W. McGuire (Eds.), *The collected works of C. G. Jung* (CW 16). Princeton, NJ: Princeton University Press.

Jung, C. G. (1946). The psychology of transference. In H. Read, M. Fordham, G. Adler, & W. McGuire (Eds.), *The collected works of C. G. Jung* (CW 16). Princeton, NJ: Princeton University Press.

Jung, C. G. (1951). Fundamental questions of psychotherapy. In H. Read, M. Fordham, G. Adler, & W. McGuire (Eds.), *The collected works of C. G. Jung* (CW 16). Princeton, NJ: Princeton University Press.

Jung, C. G. (1961). *Memories, dreams and reflections.* New York: Vintage.

Jung, C. G. (1973). Four archetypes. In R. F. C. Hull (Trans.) *Bollingen Series*XX (pp. 7–14) Princeton: Princeton University Press.

Jung, C. G. (1982). *Aspects of the feminine*. Princeton, NJ: Princeton University Press.

Jung, C. G. (1989). *Memories, dreams and reflections*. New York: Vintage. (Original work published 1963)

Katz, E., et al. (2000). *The papers of Margaret Sanger* (Columbia, S.C.: Model Editions Partnership, 1999). Electronic version. http://adh.sc.edu.

Kalter, S. (1984). *The complete book of* M.A.S.H. New York: Abrams.

Kearns-Goodwin, D. (1994). *No ordinary time: Franklin and Eleanor Roosevelt: The home front in World War II*. New York: Simon & Schuster.

Keegan, L. (1988). The history and future of healing. In B. M. Dossey, L. Keegan, & C. E. Guzzeta (Eds.), *Holistic nursing: A handbook for practice* (2nd ed., pp. 57–75). Gaithersberg, MD: Aspen.

Keegan, L. (1994). *The nurse as healer*. Albany, NY: Delmar.

Keller, H. (1902). *Helen Keller: The story of my life*. New York: Signet.

Kelly, L. Y., & Joel, L. A. (1995). *Dimensions of professional nursing* (7th ed.). McGraw-Hill: New York.

Kerenyi, K. (1959). *Asklepios, archetypal image of the physician's existence*. New York: Pantheon.

Kesey, K. (1996). *One flew over the cuckoo's nest*. New York: Penguin. (Original work published 1962).

King, S. (1996). *The green mile: The complete serial novel*. New York: Pocket Books.

Krieger, D. (1979). *The therapeutic touch: How to use your hands to heal*. Englewood Cliffs, NJ: Prentice-Hall.

Krieger, D. (1981). *Foundations for holistic health nursing practices: The renaissance nurse*. Philadelphia: Lippincott.

Krippner, S. (1988). Shamans: The first healers. In G. Doore (Ed.), *Shaman's path: Healing growth and empowerment* (pp 101–114). Boston: Shambala.

Lader, L., & Meltzer, M. (1969). *Margaret Sanger: Pioneer of birth control.* New York: Crowell.

Laub, D., & Podell, D. (1995). Art and trauma. *International Journal of Psychoanalysis*, 76 (12), 991–1005

Lefkowitz, M. R., & Fant, M. B. (1982). *Women's life in Greece and Rome*. Baltimore: Johns Hopkins.

Leppanen-Montgomery, C. (1996) The care-giving relationship: Paradoxical and transcendent aspects. *Alternative Therapies*, 2 (2), 52–57.

Levine, P., & Frederick, A. (1997). *Walking the tiger: Healing trauma*. Berkeley, CA: North Atlantic.

Lewis, S. (1927). *Elmer Gantry*. New York: Harcourt, Brace & World.

Lindemans, M. F. (2000). *The coming of medicine*. Encyclopedia Mythica. http://www.pantheon.org/.

Lipson, J. G., Dibble, S. L., & Minarik, P. A. (1996). *Culture and nursing care: A pocket guide*. San Francisco: UCSF Nursing Press.

Lumby, J. (1998). Transforming nursing through reflective practice. In C. Johns & D. Freshwater (Eds.), *Transforming nursing through reflective practice*. (pp. 91–103). London: Blackwell Science.

Madrid, M. (1994). Participating in the dying process. In M. Madrid and E. A. M. Barrett (Eds.), *Rogers' scientific art of nursing practice*. (pp. 91–100). New York : NLN.

Madrid, M., and Barrett, E. A. M. (Eds.). (1994). *Rogers' scientific art of nursing practice* (pp. 91–100). New York : NLN.

Madrid, M., & Smith, D. W. (1994). Becoming literate in the science of unitary human beings. In M. Madrid & E. A. M. Barrett (Eds.), *Rogers' scientific art of nursing practice*. New York: NLN.

Mandela, N. (1994). *The long walk to freedom*. New York: Little, Brown.

Martin, J. (2000). *A look back at Patty Hearst*. ABCNEWS.com.

Maslow, A. (1969). Various meanings of transcendence. *Journal of Transpersonal Psychology*, 1, 56–66.

Masson, M. (1985). *A pictorial history of nursing*. Twickenham, Middlesex, UK: Hamlyn.

May, R. (1985). The wounded healer. In *Perpectives in Nursing* 1985–1987 (pp. 3–11). New York: NLN.

May, R. (1989). The empathetic relationship: A foundation of healing. In R. Carlson and B. Shield (Eds.), *Healers on healing* (pp. 108–110). New York: Penguin Putnam.

McFarlane A. C., & van der Kolk, B. (1996). Trauma and its challenge to society. In B. van der Kolk, A. C. McFarlane, & L.Weisaeth, (Eds.), *Traumatic stress: The effects of overwhelming experience on mind, body and society* (pp. 24–46). New York: Guilford.

McLynn, F. (1996). *Carl Gustav Jung*. New York: St. Martin's Press.

McGlone, M. E. (1990). Healing the spirit. *Holistic Nursing Practice*, 4 (4), 77–84.

McKivergin, M. (1999) The nurse as an instrument of healing. In B. Montgomery-Dossey, L. Keegan, & C. E. Guzzetta (Eds.), *Holistic nursing: A handbook for practice*. (3rd ed., pp. 207–227). Gaithersberg, MD: Aspen.

McNiff, S. (1992). *Art as medicine* Boston: Shambala.

Meier, C. A. (1967). *Ancient incubation and modern psychotherapy*. Evanston, IL: Northwestern University Press.

Mellors, M., Riley, T., & Erlen, J. (1997). HIV, self-transcendence and quality of life. *Journal of the Association of Nurses in AIDS Care*, 8, 59–69.

Mentgen, J. (1996). The clinical practice of healing touch. In D. Hover-Kramer, J. Mentgen, & S. Scandrett-Hibdon (1996). *Healing Touch: A resource for health professionals* (pp. 155–165). Albany, NY: Delmar.

Micrsoft® Encarta® Online Encyclopedia (2000). *Arthurian legend*.

Micrsoft® Encarta® Online Encyclopedia (2000). *Eleanor Roosevelt*.

Micrsoft® Encarta® Online Encyclopedia (2000). *Holy Grail*.

Miles, M. W. (1993). The evolution of countertransference and its applicability to nursing. *Perspectives in Psychiatric Care*, 29 (4), 13–20.

Miller, G. D., & Baldwin, D. C. (1987). Implications of the wounded healer paradigm for the use of self in therapy. In M. Baldwin (Ed.), *The use of self in therapy* (pp. 139–151). Binghamton, NY: Haworth.

Montgomery-Dossey, B. M. (1998). Florence Nightingale: Her Crimean fever and chronic illness. *Journal of Holistic Nursing*, 16 (2), 168–196.

Montgomery-Dossey, B. M. (2000). *Florence Nigthengale: Mystic, visionary, healer.* Springhouse, PA: Springhouse.

Montgomery-Dossey, B., & Guzzeta, C. E. (2000). Holistic nursing practice. In B. Montgomery-Dossey, L. Keegan, & C. E. Guzzeta, (Eds.), *Holistic nursing: A Handbook for practice* (3rd ed., pp. 5–33). Gaithersberg, MD: Aspen.

Morton, A. (1998). *Diana: Her true story.* New York: Pocket Books.

Morwessel, N. J. (1994). Developing an effective pattern appraisal to guide nursing care of children with heart variations and their families. In M. Madrid & E. A. M. Barrett (Eds.), *Rogers' scientific art of nursing practice* (pp. 147–161). New York: NLN.

Muff, J. (Ed.).(1988 a). *Women's issues in nursing: Socialization, sexism and stereotyping.* Prospect Heights, IL: Waveland. (Original work published 1982)

Murphy, A. (1988). *To hell and back.* Cutchogue, NY: Buccaneer. (Original work published 1949).

Myss, C. (1996). *Anatomy of the spirit: The seven stages of power and healing.* New York: Three Rivers.

Myss, C. (1997). *Why people don't heal and how they can.* New York: Harmony.

Newman, M. (1986). *Health as expanding consciousness.* St. Louis: Mosby.

Newman, M. (1990). Shifting to higher consciousness. In M. E. Parker (Ed.), *Nursing theories in practice* (pp. 129–140). New York: NLN.

Newman, M. (1995) *Health as expanding consciousness* (2nd ed.). St. Louis: Mosby.

Nightingale, F. (1859). *Notes on nursing: What it is and what it is not.* London: Harrison.

Noer, D. M. (1993). *Healing the wounds: Overcoming the trauma of layoffs and revitalizing downsized organizations.* San Francisco: Josey Bass.

Nouwen, H. (1972). *The wounded healer.* New York: Image.

Olasov-Rothbaum, B., & Foa, E. B. (1996). Cognitive-behavioral therapy for Posttraumatic Stress Disorder. In B. van der Kolk, A. C. McFarlane, & L.Weisaeth (Eds.), *Traumatic stress: The effects of overwhelming experience on mind, body and society* (pp. 491–509). New York: Guilford.

Ondaatje, M. (1992). *The English patient.* New York: Vintage.

Original Bach® Flower Essences, (1999). *Bach Flower Essences™ for the family.* Oxfordshire, UK: Original Bach® Flower Essences.

Osteopathy Canada (1998). *Osteopathic Philosophy.* http://osteopathycanada.tripod.com/techniques.html.

Ouspensky, P. D. (1981). *The psychology of man's possible evolution.* New York: Vintage.

Parada, C. (1997) *Genealogical guide to Greek mythology.* Jonsered, Sweden: Astroms.

Parnell, L. (1997). *Transforming trauma: EMDR®: The revolutionary new therapy for freeing the mind, clearing the body and opening the heart.* New York: Norton.

Parse, R. R. (1987). *Nursing science: Major paradigms, theories and critiques.* Philadelphia: Saunders.

Parse, R. R. (1992). Human becoming: Parse's theory of nursing. *Nursing Science Quarterly, 5* 35–42.

Patterson, J. G., & Zderad, L. T. (1988). *Humanistic nursing.* New York: NLN.

Pearlman, L., & Saakvitne, K. (1995). *Trauma and the therapist: Countertransference and vicarious traumatization in psychotherapy with incest survivors.* New York: Norton.

Perera, S. B. (1981). *Descent to the goddess: A way of initiation for women.* Toronto: Inner City.

Pert, C. B. (1997) *Molecules of emotion: The science behind body-mind medicine.* New York: Touchstone.

"Phoenix (mythology)," Microsoft® Encarta® Online Encyclopedia 2000.

Pickering, G. (1974). *Creative malady: Illness in the lives and minds of Charles Darwin, Florence Nightingale, Mary Baker Eddy, Sigmund Freud, Marcel Proust and Elizabeth Barrett Browning.* New York: Oxford.

Pinkola-Estes, C. (1992). *Women who run with wolves: Myths and stories of the wild woman archetype.* New York: Ballantine.

Porter, R. (1997). *The greatest benefit to mankind: A medical history of humanity.* Norton: New York.

Quinn, J. (1999). Transpersonal caring and healing. In B. Montgomery-Dossey, L. Keegan, & C. E. Guzzetta (Eds.), *Holistic nursing: A handbook for practice* (3rd ed., pp. 37–48). Gaithersberg, MD: Aspen.

Rand, W. L. (1998). *Reiki: The healing touch: First and second degree manual.* Southfield, MI: Vision.

Reed, P. (1991a). Toward a theory of self-transcendence: Deductive transformation using developmental theories. *Advances in Nursing Science, 13,* 64–77.

Reed, P. (1991b). Self-transcendence and mental health in oldest-old adults. *Nursing Research, 40,* 1–7.

Reed, P. (1996). Transcendence: Formulating nursing perspectives. *Nursing Science Quarterly, 9* (1), 2–4.

Reis, P. (1991). Through the goddess: A woman's way of healing. New York: Continuum.

Remen, N. R. (1993). Wholeness. *Bill Moyer's healing and the mind.* New York: Doubleday.

Remen, N., May, R., Young, D., & Berland, W. (1985). The wounded healer. *Saybrook Review, 5* (1), 84–93.

Reverby, S. (1987). *Ordered to care: The dilemma of American nursing, 1850–1945.* New York: Cambridge University Press.

Roberts, J. L. (1986). *Cliff's notes on Conrad's Lord Jim.* Lincoln, NE: Cliff's Notes.

Rogers, C. (1980). *A way of being.* Boston: Houghton Mifflin.

Rogers, M. E. (1990). Nursing science of unitary, irreducible human beings: Update 1990. In E. A. M. Barrett (Ed.), *Visions of Rogers' science based nursing* (pp. 5–11). New York: NLN.

Rogers, M. E. (1992). Nursing science and the space age. *Nursing Science Quarterly, 5* (1), 27–34.

Roosevelt, E. (1960). *You learn by living.* Westminster: Knox.

Rose, G. (1995). *Necessary illusion: Art as "witness."* New York: International University Press.

Rose, H. J. (1960). *A handbook of Greek mythology: Including its extension to Rome.* New York: Dutton.

Rossman, M. (1989). Illness as an opportunity for healing. In R. Carlson & B. Shield (Eds.), *Healers on healing.* (pp. 78–81). New York: Penguin Putnam.

Rutter, P. (1995). Lot's wife, Sabina Spielrein and Anita Hill: A Jungian meditation on sexual boundary abuse and recovery of lost voices. In J. C. Gonsiorek (Ed.), *Breach of trust: Sexual exploitation by health care professionals and clergy* (pp. 75–80). Thousand Oaks, CA: Sage.

Saakvitne, K. W., & Pearlman, L. A. (1996). *Transforming the pain: A workbook on vicarious traumatization.* New York: Norton.

Sahlman, R. (2000). Harriet Tubman. *Spectrum Home and School Magazine.* [http://www.in-cwell.com/Spectrum.html] © Inc.Well DMG. Ltd.

Sandner, D. (1979). *Navaho symbols of healing.* New York: Harcourt Brace Jovanovich.

Sanger, M. (1938). *Margaret Sanger: An autobiography.* New York: Norton.

Scandrett-Hibdon, S. (1996). The history of energy-oriented healing. In D. Hover-Kramer, J. Mentgen, & S. Scandrett-Hibdon. *Healing touch: A resource for health professionals* (pp. 11–25). Albany, NY: Delmar.

Scarborough, J. (1969). *Roman medicine: Aspects of Greek and Roman life.* Ithaca, NY: Cornell University Press.

Schön, D. A. (1983). *The reflective practitioner: How professionals think in action.* New York: Basic Books.

Schaub, B., & Schaub, R. (1997). *Healing addictions.* Albany, NY: Delmar.

Schulz, M. L. (1998). *Awakening intuition: Using your mind-body network for insight and healing.* New York: Three Rivers Press.

Scully, M. (1995). Viktor Frankl at ninety: An interview. *First Things,* 4, 39–43.

Sedgwick, D. (1994). *The wounded healer: Countertransference from a Jungian perspective.* London: Routeledge.

Selanders, L. C. (1998). Florence Nightingale: The social impact of feminist values nursing. *Journal of Holistic Nursing,* 16 (2), 227–243.

Selyé, H. (1974). *Stress without distress.* New York: Signet.

Shalev, A. Y. (1996). Stress versus traumatic stress: From acute homeostatic reactions to chronic psychopathology. In B. van der Kolk, A. C. McFarlane, & L. Weisaeth (Eds.), *Traumatic stress: The effects of overwhelming experience on mind, body and society* (pp. 77–101). New York: Guilford.

Shearer, R., & Davidhizar, R. (1995). Hidden scars: Post traumatic stress disorder. *Nursing Connections,* 8 (1), 55–63.

Sheffer, M. (1988). *Bach Flower Therapy: Theory and practice.* Rochester, VT: Healing Arts.

Siegel, B. (1991). *Faithful friend: The story of Florence Nightingale.* New York: Scholastic.

Siegel, B. S. (1986). *Love, medicine and miracles.* New York: Harper & Row.

Simonton, O. C. (1989). The harmony of health. In R. Carlson & B. Shield (Eds.), *Healers on healing* (pp. 48–52). New York: Penguin Putnam.

Simonton, S. M. (1984). *The healing family: The Simonton approach for families facing illness.* New York: Bantam.

Skillings, L. (1992). Perceptions and feelings of nurses about horizontal violence as an expression of oppressed group behavior. *NLN Publications,* 14–2504 (167–185). New York: NLN.

Small, J. (1990). *Therapists of the future: Transformers: Personal transformation: The way through.* Marina del Ray, CA: DeVorss.

Smith, A. W. (1988). *Grandchildren of alcoholics: Another generation of co-dependency.* Deerfield Beach, FL: Health Communications.

Smith, D. (1999). *Being a wounded healer: How to heal ourselves while we are healing others.* Madison, WI: Psycho-Spiritual.

Smith, M. C. (1992). Nursing as metaphor. *Nursing Science Quarterly*, 5 (2), 48–49.

Snow, C., & Willard, D. (1989). *I'm dying to take care of you: Nurses and codependence: Breaking the cycles*. Redmond, WA: Professional Counselor Books.

Sohn, T., & Sohn, R. (1996). AMMA *therapy: A complete textbook of oriental bodywork and medical principles*. Rochester, VT: Healing Arts.

Stein, M. (1987). Looking backward: Archetypes in reconstruction. In N. Schwartz-Salant & M. Stein (Eds.), *Archetypal processes in psychotherapy* (pp. 197–208). Willmette, IL: Chiron.

Sterling, P., & Logan, R. (1967). *Four took freedom*. New York: Zenith.

Steppingstones, Inc. (1999) *Bill and Lois' Story*. http://wwwsteppingstones.org/.

Stewart, G. (1990). *Great mysteries: Alternative healing: Opposing viewpoints*. San Diego: Greenhaven.

Stewart, J. B. (1999) *Blind eye: The terrifying story of a doctor who got away with murder*. New York: Simon & Schuster.

Stiles, K. A. (1997). Being there: The healing power of presence. *Alternative and Complementary Therapies*, 4, 133–139.

Summers, C. (1992)a. Nursing stress: Burnout or PTSD. *Revolution*, 1, 40–46.

Summers, C. (1992)b. *Caregiver, caretaker: From dysfunctional to authentic service on nursing*. Mt. Shasta, CA: Commune-a-Key.

Swirsky, J. (1990). The psychology of abuse. In L. Gasparis & J. Swirsky (Eds.), *Nurse abuse: Impact and revolution*. New York: Power.

Symes, L. (1995). Post traumatic stress: An evolving concept. *Archives of Psychiatric Nursing*, IX (4), 195–202.

Taylor, B. (1998). Locating a phenomenological perspective of reflective nursing and midwifery practice by contrasting interpretive and critical reflection. In C. Johns & D. Freshwater (Eds.), *Transforming nursing through reflective practice* (pp. 134–150). London: Blackwell Science.

"Theresa of Lisieux, Saint," Microsoft® Encarta® Online Encyclopedia 2000 http://encarta.msn.com©

Thoma, I. K. (1990). The Door to the Possible, Sutdiok@ma.ultranet.com.

Thomsen, R. (1975). *Bill W*. New York: Harper & Row.

Titchener, E. B. (1912). The schema of introspection. *American Journal of Psychology*, 23, 485–508.

Tomb, D. A. (1994). The phenomenology of Post-traumatic stess disorder. *Psychiatric Clinics of North America*, 17(2), 237–250.

Topalian, E. (1984). *Margaret Sanger*. New York: Watts.

Upchurch, S. (1999). Self transcendence and activities of daily living: The woman with the pink slippers. *Journal of Holistic Nursing*, 17 (3), 251–266.

Upledger, J. (1989). Self-discovery and self-healing. In R. Carlson and B. Shield (Eds.), *Healers on healing* (pp. 67–72). New York: Penguin Putnam.

van der Kolk, B. (1996). The body keeps score: Approaches to the psychobiology of Posttraumatic stress disorder. In B. van der Kolk, A.C. McFarlane, & L. Weisaeth, (Eds.), *Traumatic stress: The effects of overwhelming experience on mind, body and society* (pp. 3–23). New York: Guilford.

van der Kolk, B. (1998). The psychology and psychobiology of developmental trauma. In A. Stoudemire (Ed.). *Human behavior: An introduction for medical students* (pp. 383–399). New York: Lippincott-Raven.

van der Kolk, B. (2000). The assessment and treatment of complex PTSD. In R. Yahuda (Ed.), *Traumatic stress* (pp. 1–20). Washington, DC: American Psychiatric Press.

van der Kolk, B., & McFarlane, A. C. (1996). The black hole of trauma. In B. van Der Kolk, A.C. McFarlane, & L. Weisaeth (Eds.), *Traumatic Stress: The effects of overwhelming experience on mind, body and society* (pp. 214– 241). New York: Guilford.

van der Kolk, B., McFarlane, A. C., & van der Hart (1996). A general approach to treatment of Posttraumatic stress disorder. In B. van der Kolk, A. C. McFarlane, & L.Weisaeth (Eds.), *Traumatic stress: The effects of overwhelming experience on mind, body and society.* (pp. 417–440). New York: Guilford.

van der Post, L. (1975). *Jung and the story of our time.* New York: Random House.

Vaughn, F. E. (1979). Transpersonal dimensions of psychotherapy. *Re-Vision,* 2 (1), 26–29.

Wade, G. H. (1998). A concept analysis of personal transformation. *Journal of Advanced Nursing,* 28 (4), 713–719.

Wade, N. (2000, November 7). Teaching the body to heal itself. *The New York Times,* pp. F1, F8.

Walker, A. (1982). *The color purple.* New York: Harcourt Brace Jovanovich.

Wallace, L. (1978). *Ben-Hur: A tale of the Christ.* New York: Bonanza. (Original work published 1880).

Watson, J. (1987). Nursing on the caring edge: Metaphorical vignettes. *Advances in Nursing Science,* 10 (1), 10–18.

Watson, J. (1988). *Nursing: Human science and human caring: A theory of nursing.* New York: NLN.

Watson, J. (1999a). *Postmodern nursing and beyond.* New York: Churchill Livingstone.

Watson, J. (1999b). Relationship centered caring. Keynote Speech Department of Veterans Affairs, New York Harbor Health Care System November 4, 1999. The Second Symposium on Patient Centered Care.

Weil, A. (1983). *Health and healing: Understanding conventional and alternative medicine.* Boston: Houghton Mifflin.

Wendler, M. C. (1996). Understanding healing: A conceptual analysis. *Journal of Advanced Nursing,* 24, 836–842.

West, M. L., & Keller, A. E. (1991). Parentification of the child: A case study of Bowlby's compulsive care-giving attachment pattern. *American Journal of Psychotherapy,* 45 (3), 425–431.

Whan, M. (1987). Chiron's wound: Some reflections on the wounded healer. In N. Schwartz-Salant & M. Stein (Eds.), *Archetypal processes in psychotherapy* (pp. 197–209). Willmette, IL: Chiron.

Whorton, J. C. (1988). Patient, heal thyself: Popular health reform movements as unorthodox medicine. In N. Gevitz (Ed.), *Other healers: Unorthodox medicine in America* (pp. 52–81). Baltimore: Johns Hopkins.

Whitfield, C. (1991). Co-Dependence: Healing the human condition. Deerfield Beach, FL: Health Communications.

Whitfield, C. (1995). Memory and abuse: Remembering and healing the effects of trauma. Deerfield Beach, FL: Health Communications.

Wiesen-Cook, B. (1992). Eleanor Roosevelt, Vol. 1: 1884–1932. New York: Viking Penguin.

Wilbur, K. (1993). The spectrum of consciousness. Wheaton, IL: Quest.

Wilkinson, J. (1999). Implementing reflective practice. Nursing Standard, 13 (21), 36–40.

Willis, P. (1999). Looking for what it's really like: Phenomenology in reflective practice. Studies in Continuing Education, 21 (10), 91–112.

Wilson, A. (2000) Aeneas: The underworld. The classics page. www.classicspage.com.

Wilson, L. (1979). Lois remembers: Memoirs of the co-founder of Al-Anon and wife of the co-founder of Alcoholics Anonymous. Virginia Beach, VA: Al-Anon Family Group Headquarters.

Woititz, J. (1985). Struggle for intimacy. Pompano Beach, FL: Health Communications.

Wolinsky, S. (1993). The dark side of the inner child: The next step. Fall Village, CT: Bramble.

Wolinsky, S., & Gordon, M. (1986). Trances people live: Healing approaches in quantum psychology. Fall Village, CT: Bramble.

Woods-Smith, D. (1994). Viewing polio survivors through violet tinted glasses. In M. Madrid and E. A. M. Barrett (Eds.), Rogers' scientific art of nursing practice (pp. 141–144). New York: NLN.

Woodman, M. (1990). Addiction to perfection: The roots of compulsive behavior and the need for spiritual fulfillment [Audiocassette]. Boston: Shambala.

Wright, S. G. (1986). Building and using a model of nursing. London: Arnold.

Wundt, W. (1897). Outlines of psychology. Leipzig: Engelmann.

Young A. (1993), AMMA therapy: A holistic approach to chronic fatigue. Journal of Holistic Nursing, 11 (2), 172–182.

Zand, J., Spreen, A., & LaValle, J. (1999). Smart medicine for healthier living: A practical A–Z reference to natural and conventional treatment for adults. Garden City Park, NY: Avery.

Zimbalist, S. (Producer), & Wyler, W. (Director). (1959). Ben-Hur [Videocassette]. Available from MGM/UA Home Video, Inc., 1000 Washington Boulevard, Culver City, CA, 90232.

Zukav, G. (1989) The seat of the soul. New York: Simon & Schuster.

INDEX

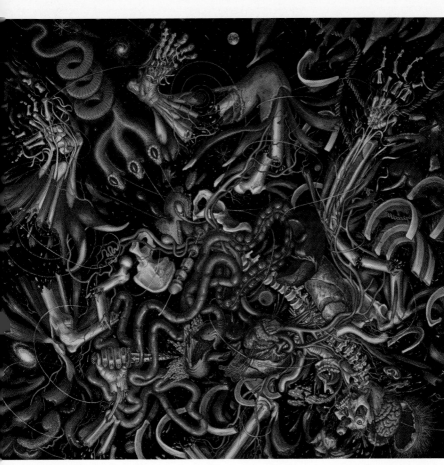

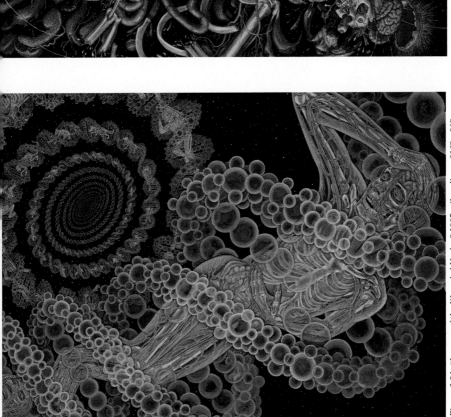

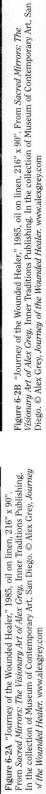

Figure 6-2B "Journey of the Wounded Healer," 1985, oil on linen, 216" x 90". From *Sacred Mirrors: The Visionary Art of Alex Grey*, Inner Traditions Publishing. In the collection of Museum of Contemporary Art, San Diego. © Alex Grey, *Journey of the Wounded Healer*. www.alexgrey.com

Figure 6-2A "Journey of the Wounded Healer," 1985, oil on linen, 216" x 90". From *Sacred Mirrors: The Visionary Art of Alex Grey*, Inner Traditions Publishing. In the collection of Museum of Contemporary Art, San Diego. © Alex Grey, *Journey of the Wounded Healer*. www.alexgrey.com

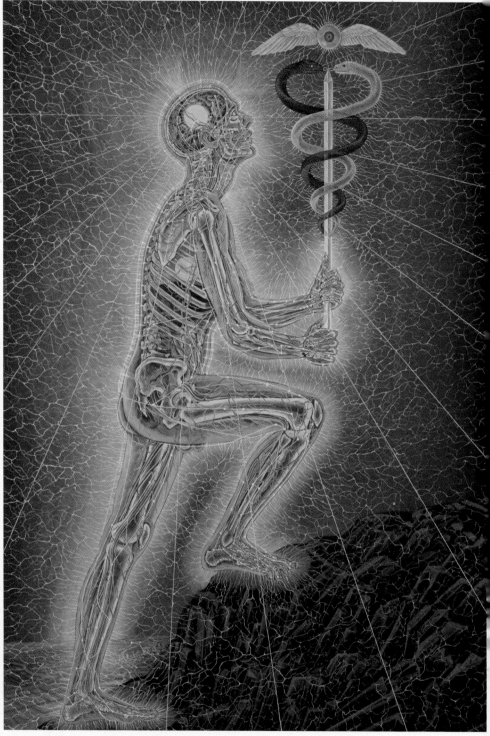

Figure 6-2C "Journey of the Wounded Healer," 1985, oil on linen, 216" x 90". From *Sacred Mirrors: The Visionary Art of Alex Grey,* Inner Traditions Publishing. In the collection of Museum of Contemporary Art, San Diego. © Alex Grey, *Journey of the Wounded Healer.* www.alexgrey.com